Easy Sugar Break-Up

First published in 2007 as *The Craving Cure* and now includes new, updated material, including information on cutting-edge tools such as medical grade CBD oil and recipes.

Published by Lisa Hagan Books 2019

www.lisahaganbooks.com

Powered by

SHADOW TEAMS

Cover design and interior layout by Simon Hartshorne

EASY SUGAR BREAK-UP

Break the Habits and Addictions That Control You

RENA GREENBERG

Founder of Wellness Seminars INC

Foreword by Bernie Siegel, M.D.

This book is dedicated with deep love, appreciation and gratitude, to my dear husband, Barry, for his ever-deepening love and support, to my amazing Mother, and to my two beautiful daughters, Crystal and Jessie, who are the light of my life.

Contents

Foreword

Bernie Siegel, M.D.

What does every woman or man want? What do we all crave in this life? We all want a life of our own and not a life imposed upon us. The sad part is that when we give up our healthy and true desires, we lose our lives and our cravings become self-destructive and depersonalizing.

When our relationship with life becomes unhealthy, so does our relationship with food. Separating one's life from one's desires leads to unhealthy cravings and addictions. Self-destruction replaces self-esteem, and we seek foods that will give us the feelings we no longer can experience and artificial means of providing ourselves and our bodies with temporary relief from our losses.

What we all need to do is wake up, reclaim our lives and desires, and not deny ourselves what we are entitled to: a life of our own. We need to choose life and accept and love ourselves. Rena Greenberg's book can help you to find self-love and the intention necessary to restore a healthy lifestyle with a craving for life. Through her experience and wisdom, she is able to help you find the inspiration necessary to use the information she provides.

People whose lives are being destroyed by unhealthy cravings are not stupid. They know what they are doing is not good for them, but they do not have the determination necessary to be reborn and act like the person they want to be. It is no accident that the term *born-again* comes up so frequently in the lives of those who are awakened by addictions, diseases, and disasters and find new meaning in their lives.

This book can help you to turn a curse into a blessing, but you must be ready to do it. No one can do it for you. Others can only coach you. You must be ready to show up for practice and rehearse being the person you have created as your new role model. It is crazy, but people take better care of their pets than they do of themselves. We are asking you to step forward and love yourself. Why is that so hard to do? Your past is the culprit. So start now: abandon your past and begin a new life with *Easy Sugar Break-Up*.

To do this you must trust yourself and your feelings and be ready to forgive yourself when you lose your way. You are a work in progress and can always touch up or redo things if you do not create the work of art you intended. It is time to dump the guilt, shame, and blame and move into faith, hope, and love as your motivators. *Easy Sugar Break-Up* can guide you through the steps necessary to create the new you. What you need is to care about yourself and be willing to look within and deal with the destructive messages and words that are driving your cravings.

The solution lies in creating and unifying a healthy mind and body. Contained in this book are the directions that can help you to heal both the emotional and physical aspects of your life. When the practical and spiritual become one, we crave health through love. So my prescription for you is to read *Easy Sugar Break-Up* and heal yourself and your life.

Introduction

Are you constantly thinking about the foods that you are or aren't going to eat? Or the substances that you are aren't going to consume? Do you have "favorite" foods or combinations of foods that you feel compelled to go out of your way to eat? Are there particular types of foods or substances that you just can't live without? Do you have certain rituals with food or other substances—such as alcohol or drugs--prescription or otherwise—that you revolve your life around? Have you eliminated a category of food only to substitute excessive consumption of another category, for example eliminating caffeine and then drinking more alcohol or eating more sugar or snack food instead?

Do you stick to your "diet" all day long only to find yourself raiding the refrigerator at night? When you try to stop eating sugary foods or drinking alcohol or caffeine, do you experience withdrawal? If you answered yes to the majority of these questions, then it is very likely that you have an unhealthy relationship with food (or any substance) that can be labeled an addiction.

Addiction may seem like a strong word. However, the definition of addiction is "a state of physiological or psychological dependence on a drug liable to have a damaging effect." Sugar is a drug you have undoubtedly become dependent upon, in its various forms. It's likely that you are already aware of the devastating consequences sugar, along with caffeine and alcohol, is having on your body. Although sugar and simple carbohydrates give you a short-term boost in energy and mood, over the long run over-indulging in sugar damages all your bodily systems. The overconsumption of sugar and simple, processed carbohydrates can lead to overweight, fatigue, mood swings, depression, anxiety, headaches, irritable bowel syndrome, heart disease, dental carries, arthritis, autoimmune disease, candidiasis, diabetes, and stroke.

Craving sugar in the form of chocolate or sweets; white flour products such as bread, cereal, pretzels and pasta; french fries, popcorn, and chips; alcohol; or stimulants such as caffeine and diet pills may seem harmless. After all, a craving is nothing more than a strong desire or yearning. However, the real issue is, where does that craving lead? Does it lead to the painful experience of obsessing about food or stimulants—waiting for your next fix? Do you sometimes feel that your food or stimulant cravings are taking over your life? The line between craving and addiction is very thin.

If you are unhappy with your relationship with food, caffeine or alcohol, if you find yourself eating foods that you know are harmful to you or cause you to feel bad either psychologically or physically, or if you feel completely out of control around food (or any other substance), then this book is for you. Whether your weakness is a daily cocktail after work, a bag of chips or a bowl of popcorn in the afternoon, or a cup of coffee and a muffin in the morning, or smoking a joint or cigarette after work, your regular indulging could be setting you up for insatiable cravings.

Sugar, alcohol, caffeine, and simple carbohydrates require minimal digestion and therefore dump sugar into the blood. This creates huge spikes and dips in your blood sugar due to the excess insulin that is secreted, adrenal exhaustion from the constant release of hormones, and a depletion of necessary "feel-good" brain chemicals. This chain of events translates into extreme fluctuations in your mood and energy level. That's when that insatiable urge for your next dose of sugar or stimulant, in any form, overtakes you.

Food cravings are caused and perpetuated by five possible factors:

- **Low blood sugar or physical hunger.** If you are not eating regularly, not eating enough food, skipping breakfast, or eating simple carbohydrates that are turning into sugar quickly in your bloodstream, then it is likely that your cravings are the result of hunger caused by dips in your blood sugar.

- **Malnutrition.** Your body is simply not getting the nutrients it needs, so you keep putting food in your mouth in a vain attempt to give your system the essential vitamins, minerals, cannabinoids and phytonutrients it requires to survive. You are eating as a way to correct an intrinsic nutritional deficiency or a metabolic imbalance.

- **Sensitivities.** Certain foods may not agree with you or may cause a symptomatic reaction, such as fatigue or moodiness. Ironically, until you discover the culprit, your body will continue to yearn for the very item that is creating the allergenic response. The body is tricked into thinking that the desired food offers a relief from symptoms, when in reality it is the cause.

- **Unresolved emotional issues.** We eat, smoke, drink or pop pills as a way to stuff sadness, anger, guilt. boredom, or loneliness or to give ourselves nurturing, love, safety, and comfort.

- **Eating to reduce stress.** Using food, drugs or alcohol to cope when overwhelmed by life's details may be feeding your addiction to unhealthy foods. Even not drinking enough water—and allowing yourself to become dehydrated—can be a source of physical stress. It's not uncommon to overeat or reach for a stimulant in an effort to self-soothe and balance brain chemicals.

If you are unhappy with the results your food and lifestyle choices are having on your body, it's time to make a change. If you could simply make an outer change such as eating more vegetables, or getting rid of your end of the day cocktails, you would. However, how many times have you set such goals for yourself only to sabotage yourself shortly thereafter? It's important to understand that the reason for your previous failure has nothing to do with willpower, motivation, or intelligence. Intellectually, you are well aware of the perils of living a life fueled by craving for sugary foods or stimulating substances. You know that your lifestyle and overconsumption of simple and processed carbohydrates is wreaking havoc on your endocrine and nervous systems.

The challenge you face is that you are driven to perpetuate your destructive behavior by the incessant seeking of pleasure from within. Until you connect with the deeper parts of yourself—within your heart, where your true resources lie—you are destined to continue your self-sabotaging behavior. The only way to have complete freedom from the painful, seemingly never-ending cycle of sugar, carbohydrate, alcohol and stimulant cravings is to finally learn to fulfill that drive for pleasure, not by gratifying the ever-changing desires of the personality or self, but by going deeper within to the wisdom of your greater heart and soul. I refer to this place as your core, or your essence, behind the constant chatter of the conscious, limited aspect of your mind. Once you harness the vast power within—which is often out of your day-to-day awareness, compulsively reaching for sugar will become a thing of the past. Your fear of withdrawal will pale beside your ability to witness your greater capacity to live a fuller, more fulfilling life despite the emotional ups and downs that are a part of life.

I speak from personal experience when I say that it is absolutely possible to change the way you think about food and be free from food, sweets, alcohol, caffeine and drug addiction forever. I personally was addicted to sugar, caffeine, alcohol, a variety of substances and almost all simple, processed carbohydrates over twenty years ago. I craved stimulating foods or substances and could not imagine going one day without them, let alone eliminating them forever. Truly, my life felt empty if I wasn't focused on food, alcohol or caffeine in one way or another. I overate and drank alcohol when I was socializing, and I overate and drank excessive coffee when I was alone. I ate because I was happy, sad, stressed, or bored. I used stimulating foods or substances to give me energy and keep me going when I was tired, and then I used food to help me fall asleep at night. When I got together with friends, my greatest concern was where we were going to eat, drink or party.

My life took an unexpected turn when I got very sick at a young age. By my mid-twenties, I was literally facing death with an irregular heart rate of 30 beats per minute and on the verge of diabetes. Suddenly I began to feel chronically exhausted. Prior to discovering that my heart rate was so low, I went from doctor to doctor in search of a cure for my exhaustion, but was always told the same thing—no physical cause for my symptoms could be found.

One day, I walked into the emergency room, unsure if there was really anything wrong with me. To my surprise, I was whisked into the cardiac care unit and told by the chief of cardiology that I had the heart of an eighty-year-old. When I came to the realization that there was something so drastically amiss with my body and my life could end so abruptly, I stopped to take a hard look at how I was living.

The doctors knew of no cause for my condition, but I began to suspect my unhealthy lifestyle. I realized that I had been giving little thought to the food and beverages I was consuming. When I had cut back on sugar, I had increased my intake of sugar substitutes, completely oblivious to the fact that these products are filled with harmful chemicals that have a direct impact on the brain and all the bodily systems. The hidden chemicals in foods and sugar substitutes perpetuate the craving for more of the same. The processed foods industry was literally keeping me hooked on unhealthy foods that were depleting me of vital nutrients. I learned how eating empty-calorie foods actually sucks out much-needed vitamins and minerals from the body in their digestion. I also reflected on how I had used exercise in an unhealthy way, forcing myself to exude large amounts of energy to burn the abundance of calories I was taking in, even when I felt exhausted. At that time, I made a commitment to myself to do whatever it took to break free from the harmful, vicious cycle I felt trapped by.

It was only by connecting with the deeper power inside my own heart and soul that I hadn't been consciously aware of, behind all the pictures and voices that had me convinced that I needed to consume sugar or caffeine in order to be happy, that I was able to turn my health and my life around. I began to embrace my health and the precious life that I had been given. I read everything I could on nutrition and began to eat in a balanced, moderate way. I found foods I loved that would give my body sustenance and eliminate physical hunger.

I discovered the importance of incorporating healthy fat into my diet, and eating in a balanced way—meaning enough pure protein, lots of water-rich veggies and salad, balanced with just the right amount of complex carbohydrate, to feel completely satiated. I also learned the importance, psychologically, of not ever feeling like I was on a "diet" of any kind. Dieting, subconsciously, is restriction and no one wants to feel limited or deprived. Instead I realized that I could think of my new way of eating as a lifestyle that I had gladly chosen. As a result of this new way of life, my mood swings and radical shifts in energy level disappeared, and I was left feeling calmer, more peaceful, and in control of my life.

I realized the incredible power beyond the conscious mind that we can access through meditation and self-hypnosis to change the way we think about ourselves and food subconsciously. I began to study everything I could about how to tap into the power of the mind for permanent change. I received my degree in biopsychology from the City University of New York and later went on to complete certifications in hypnotherapy, energy healing and neurolinguistic programming and as a biofeedback therapist. Shortly after that, I began teaching the method I had used to turn my life around in hospitals throughout the country. Since 1989, I have helped over two hundred thousand people break their addictions to food and tobacco, lose weight, and gain health in over seventy-five medical centers. I founded Wellness Seminars, Incorporated, and began to present smoking cessation and weight-control programs using the power of hypnosis to the employees of major corporations such as Walt Disney World and Home Depot, city governments, and hospitals throughout the country.

Each of us has the power within to improve our lives beyond anything we may have imagined, when we are given the tools. *Easy Sugar Break-Up* will provide you with these tools, which include setting an effective intention, self-hypnosis, breathing, learning to love and honor yourself, physical exercise, and nutrition, including using plants such as herbs and CBD for mind-body healing.

The Two-Week Mega-Nutrition Cleanse is an easy and efficient way to help eliminate any toxins in your body that leave you feeling sluggish and wanting your next "fix" of sugar or simple, processed carbohydrate. This will address your physical urges for certain foods. At the same time, the Break-Your-Craving-State Technique will help to release you from the psychological triggers that in the past have caused you to reach for the substances that are harmful to you. Here's an overview of what you will learn.

- **Hypnosis.** Hypnosis and self-hypnosis is a way to break deep-seated patterns by changing your subconscious perceptions. All hypnosis is essentially self hypnosis, because you alone hold the power to allow new thoughts, ideas and mental movies to infiltrate your mind. The choice to change is yours, in every moment. The tools you will learn in *Easy Sugar Break-Up* offer you a way to use the same principles that make hypnotherapy so effective and allow dramatic, lasting changes to occur, but without needing to go into a formal trance.

You will learn to break out from the everyday trances you are already in and free yourself from the grip of harmful suggestions that permeate our environment, telling us that it's normal to eat processed foods, in excess, that may be toxic to our system. You can hypnotize yourself into preferring those foods that are best for you and make you feel good both inside and out—the foods that really feed and nourish your body and mind. *Easy Sugar Break-Up* will teach you how to harness the greater power within the core of your being to eliminate doubt and step into a life of true happiness, health, and control over your eating habits. Without needing to go into a formal trance, you will begin to incorporate the techniques that make hypnosis so effective—imagery, affirmations, relaxation, focused concentration, questioning belief systems—in order to create lasting change.

- **Setting your intention.** A form of self-hypnosis, setting your intention will help you make your goal so vivid and the object of your desire so real to your subconscious mind that you'll naturally begin to eliminate harmful foods and prefer healthier selections.

- **Learning to love yourself.** It may seem like indulging in rich, forbidden food is a way of giving to yourself, but when continued in excess, it's actually a form of self-abuse. Deep in your heart, your being craves love, nurturance, peace, safety, and comfort. In *Easy Sugar Break-Up*, you'll learn ways of giving to yourself, loving and honoring yourself, and filling your deeper needs without being caught in an endless cycle of cravings.

- **Breathing.** Often we reach for food as a way to gain energy or calm ourselves down. In either case, the outcome of using food in this way is most often not desirable. It's possible that what you perceive as hunger is in fact a lack of oxygen.

Your body may be crying out for this vital nutrient. It is so easy to go through the day, caught up in the demands of life, without even having conscious awareness that we are barely breathing. You'll learn easy-to-use breathing techniques that will have you both relaxed and energized— physically and mentally—leaving you in a state of peacefulness and vitality. You'll also learn how to use your breath to calm and relax yourself in times of stress, so that you no longer need to reach for unhealthy foods.

- **Physical exercise.** The importance of physical movement in maintaining a balanced state of health, free from cravings, cannot be over-estimated. You'll learn to reframe your entire perspective on exercise. Rather than experiencing exercise as a painful chore, you will learn to look forward to the pleasurable sensations of moving your body. As you find new ways to incorporate activity into your lifestyle, you'll find your focus on food as your main source of pleasure in life shift. Physical activity will become a new means to invigorate yourself and bring much-needed oxygen and other vital nutrients to all the cells of your body.

- **The Break-Your-Craving-State Technique.** The Break-Your-Craving-State Technique in Chapter 7 is the culmination of the methods to raise cellular energy naturally, increase your self-esteem and confidence, and sharpen your ability to listen to the deep wisdom of your heart outlined in Chapters 3 through 6. It's a very powerful form of self-hypnosis that allows you to bypass the critical voices of the conscious mind so that you can begin to relate to yourself in a new way. The Break-Your-

Craving-State Technique is a revolutionary method that shortcuts the entire sequence of events that occurs when you feel overcome by desire for sweet, salty, or processed, carbohydrate-rich foods. It gives you a very effective alternative to drugging yourself with these substances and ultimately creating more misery for yourself.

The Break-Your-Craving-State

This technique works on many levels to help you instantly change your inner state and make new choices that are in alignment with your deep desire to create permanent change in your health, eating habits, and your life. All aspects of yourself are employed—your mind, body, and spirit—to shift your thoughts, feelings, and behaviors to those that will lead you to the result you have been praying for. After you have learned to identify the parts of yourself that are conflicted and how to use that knowledge to achieve the goals you have set for yourself, you will be able to use the Break-Your-Craving-State Technique to engage all these levels for optimum results—a healthy, fit body and a life of happiness and peace.

- **Detox/nutrition.** I encourage you to eat the foods discussed in Chapter 8, "High-Nutrition Eating," as soon as you can. In fact, if you are motivated, it's OK to read that chapter first so that you can begin the program immediately. Why wait any longer to begin to reap the benefits of healthy, nutritious, moderate eating? You must make the commitment to leave your old eating habits and destructive ways of the past behind. At your earliest convenience, head to your local natural foods store, farmer's market, or grocery to stock up on those foods that will bring you health: water-rich, whole, unprocessed foods, healthy omega 3 fat, complex carbohydrate and pure protein. You'll find lots of ideas for preparing and combining foods for maximum enjoyment and nutritional value in this chapter. Does eating mostly water-rich, unprocessed, clean, whole food feel like a major leap to you? If so, don't despair. The Two-Week Mega-Nutrition Cleanse described in Chapter 11 will help to physically clean your body so that you actually begin to prefer health-promoting, life-giving foods. This gentle and effective approach also helps to alleviate any withdrawal symptoms you may have experienced in the past when you tried to eliminate harmful foods. By following the *Easy Sugar Break-Up* program, you'll not only discover the vast benefits of drinking lots of pure water, fresh vegetable juicing, eating healthy, whole food in a balanced way, power breathing, and physical movement, but you'll begin to look forward to this new, energizing way of life.

- **Herbal Balancing with CBD.** CBD, short for Cannabidiol, is the new buzz word. In fact, CBD is often being described as a miracle plant healer. With so much hype around CBD, it's difficult to know what's true. Can CBD be used to help break free from addiction, including incessant food cravings? The answer is, yes! However, to use CBD effectively for weight loss, health, freedom from addiction and balancing, it's essential that you understand what to look for when buying CBD. What makes CBD medical grade? CBD has so much potential to help you end your addiction to food or any other substance because a substantial aspect of addiction is the mind-body seeking relief from pain, and balance. Discover how your body's endo-cannabinoid system works and how CBD, with or without other herbs, can help your body to achieve much-needed homeostasis, in Chapter 9.

A New Source of Fulfillment

Though you may be accustomed to relating to yourself in terms of your personality, your desires, your body and appearance, your accomplishments, and your mind, you are in fact so much more than the sum of all of these parts. Inside you is a level of power, creativity, peace, joy, wisdom, love, and beauty that you may only have had rare glimpses of up until this point. The purpose of this book is to help you find these inner riches so you stop looking to food for inner fulfillment. The method is an inward journey to the core of your being, behind the outer reflections of what's happening in your life and the various parts of yourself.

Through the program outlined in this book, you will reconnect to those long-forgotten places of deep peace and personal commitment inside yourself and eliminate the sugar cravings that have kept you feeling frustrated and desperate. At the same time, you will discover how to enjoy and look forward to those foods that nourish and sustain you. You will begin to honor yourself and realize at a very deep level how precious and blessed your life really is. Your innate desire to respect your body will spring forth naturally.

Thank you for letting me share with you the tools that have changed my life. I remember what it was like to have my entire day revolve around my compulsion to eat or avoid certain foods or substances. I speak from personal experience when I say that it is absolutely possible to live life without those horrible, energy-draining cravings and the physical and mental pain that ensues. Because of my own experience, and the stories from thousands of people who have shared with me how they were able to conquer their own food and other addictions by using these tools, I am convinced that you, too, can over-come the strongest of cravings for foods, drugs or alcohol that are toxic to your system. Whether you are a daily binger, someone who can't live without your morning cappuccino and breakfast scone or a person who spends all week fantasizing about the french fries or Fettuccini Alfredo that you'll get to eat on the weekend, *Easy Sugar Break-Up* will help you to relate to yourself and food in a completely new way. It is my deepest desire and privilege to guide you on this journey.

It's true that addiction and craving are deeply rooted in the physical—hence the benefit of including CBD and high nutrition eating as part of your daily regimen, as well as giving your body a healing two week cleanse. However, in order to break free from addiction and unproductive habits, permanently, you need to shift your perceptions.

My goal is to help you stop the vicious cycle of dieting and get off the endless roller coaster of consuming addictive substances, without ever feeling deprived or denied. The key to success is realizing the vast power within your own mind.

On my PBS show, I talked about a recent study at the National Institute of Health that used brain scans in adult men and women to prove that your preferences for food and any other substance can actually change in the brain. That's exciting!

Remember breaking up with an old girlfriend or boyfriend, of younger years, and spending days, weeks or months, crying over him or her? Did you ever have the experience of looking back and realizing that if that person came back in your life now, you would have absolutely zero interest?

If you can relate, take a moment and think about what happened. It's simple: your perception shifted. I want you to know the same exact mental shift is possible with any addictive substance in your life, including food.

You can literally look at the ice-cream, beer, pills or pizza the way you would look at an old lover who you realize is no good for you—with disgust and/or disinterest. Instead of being overcome with desire for a toxin in your life, it's possible instead to feel a surge of freedom the way you might when you realize that you are done with all the pain that an old relationship caused you. The key is to realize this is your choice rather than a rejection or deprivation that is happening to you. In the same way, you can look at harmful foods and toxic substances and actually feel great about not partaking.

There's a huge difference between thinking you want something but can't have it (which is the entire premise of dieting) and realizing that you are done—finished—with putting toxic substances, on any level, into your life. I want you to never feel like you are on a diet again—which is so painful—and instead my prayer for you is a complete feeling of freedom as you realize that you are *choosing* to live your life alive, aware and healthy—mentally, physically and emotionally—and everything you do or don't put in your body supports that *decision*.

If your goal is weight loss, I encourage you to let the desire for fat loss become a side benefit. Stop white knuckling it. Aren't you done with the myriad of diets that you've already been on? Isn't it time to stop looking for that "perfect new diet" and just start tuning in to the wisdom of your body to know what your body actually needs? Imagine treating yourself with love and respect the way you would treat your newborn baby—with honor and care, rather than stuffing yourself with any substance the advertising or food industry decides to put in your path. By putting the focus on your wellness and taking actions and making choices based on your commitment to transform your health, not only is any weight loss you are seeking likely to be a side benefit, but your whole life can be transformed and taken to a new level of happiness and freedom. Thank you for taking this journey with me.

Part I. Breaking Free from Cravings

1. The Power of Intention to Break the Cravings

Chances are you picked up this book because you feel compelled to give in to unmanageable cravings for snack foods, simple, processed carbohydrates, alcohol, sweets, or stimulants. Do you feel that you are often out of control around food? Do you find yourself compulsively reaching for sugar-filled foods even when you have made a decision not to? Do you turn to food as a way to stimulate yourself or suppress what you are actually feeling?

For example, you may find yourself feeling tired, but rather than lie down and rest, you reach for chocolate. Perhaps you have a big chore ahead of you—like cleaning the house, mowing the yard, or writing an important proposal—but rather than get started, you find yourself in the kitchen, inspecting the contents of your refrigerator. Maybe you are feeling remorseful because you were a little hard on your son, but rather than have to face what you are feeling, you distract yourself by turning on the TV and munching on a bag of Cheetos. What is it that you are truly seeking?

If you are like most people, you seek to be happy, to be fulfilled, to have a vital and meaningful life. You also probably wish to avoid sickness, pain, and discomfort. These desires are innate and very positive. People have always searched for ways to make themselves feel better—from spinning around as children to discovering foods that create that little extra buzz of energy or sense of well-being. Seeking happiness outside yourself may seem like the most natural thing to do. Even though you can certainly find momentary pleasure in the foods you eat, the addictive impulses that are guiding you are slowly chipping away at the quality of your life.

You may think, too, that your favorite foods are your greatest source of pleasure or comfort. It may seem that way, but at what cost? It's amazing how much suffering we can block out to justify our desire to continue with an unhealthy addiction. Once we realize what we are truly searching for—such as love, safety, deep rest—it can be a relief because we are likely to get what we truly want only after we have the courage to break free from our old, destructive habits.

The good news is that you can have all that you desire, and most important you can be free from your sugar addiction. I define sugar addiction as the compulsion to consume sugar, simple carbohydrates, stimulating foods, or beverages containing sugar, sweeteners, caffeine, or alcohol. This means turning to these items as you would to a drug—to stimulate, sedate, or distract—and feeling compelled to eat them even when you intellectually know it's not best for you.

What Is It That You Are Craving?

Your addiction is caused by your insatiable desire to feel full and more alive. When you eat sugar and the rush of feel-good chemicals floods your bloodstream, you get the momentary pleasure you crave. Unfortunately, when your blood sugar begins to plummet as a result of the assault the glucose imposes on your bodily systems, it only causes you to desperately want more. When your behavior stems from addiction, you will never feel fulfilled in the long run. It is like being trapped in a cage, with your arm extended, seeking more of that which put you in the cage in the first place. The freedom that you seek is possible, and the strength that you need to find that freedom is within you, but it will not come through ingesting substances that are ultimately toxic to your system.

Rationally, you know that your behavior is harmful to you. If you didn't have the good fortune to discover this fact about yourself—that certain foods are poisonous to your system—your ignorance would keep you in a vicious cycle of indulging, gaining more and more weight, or having an increase in symptoms that make you feel bad, and feeling more and more trapped by the consequences of succumbing to your addictive tendencies. The pain of your compulsive behavior and the ill effect your eating style has on your physical, mental, and emotional health would be outside of your level of consciousness. You might even feel like a victim in the face of the ensuing and mounting health problems you were faced with. Food addiction (specifically sugar and simple carbohydrates) has been linked to physical ailments such as diabetes, stroke, obesity, osteoporosis, heart disease, dental cavities, arthritis, autoimmune disease, candidiasis, inflammation, kidney stones, and chronic fatigue syndrome.

Emotionally and mentally, food addiction has been linked to anxiety, depression, suicidal thoughts, hyperactivity, PMS, insomnia, irritability, and anger. Besides being a source of empty calories, sugar is a drug that upsets the entire balance and delicate workings of your body, often leading to dire consequences and a host of physical and psychological problems.

Why do you continue to eat and live in a way that is harmful to you and puts you at risk for illness or premature death? Why would you continue to reach for foods that are likely to perpetuate mood swings, fatigue, or even create a mental imbalance? Is it just because sweet foods and beverages taste so good? Yes, temptation abounds, and yet there is a much deeper reason why you are on a self-imposed roller-coaster, self-medicating with seemingly innocent and yet potentially harmful, if not lethal, substances.

Seeking Pleasure Through Food

Having a conscious knowledge of the many health risks of harmful foods and drinks may not be a strong enough deterrent to break your addiction. This is because, on some level, eating sugary foods has been pleasurable to you, and you have a perceived benefit. Perhaps this benefit is a temporary relief from the hardships in life, a feeling of camaraderie with friends, or a sudden burst in energy and feeling uplifted from fatigue or depression.

Your addiction, or habit—whether it be to rich, sugary foods or other simple carbohydrates—is fueled by your desire to achieve a certain inner state. Even though being stuffed with food feels miserable, on some level you believe it will ultimately lead you to feeling good or getting the love and happiness that you want and deserve—so you keep repeating the negative behavior. Even though drinking margaritas and eating greasy nachos leaves you feeling hungover and remorseful, you associate fun and youth with your drinking and eating sprees. Late-night binging may leave you too exhausted or spaced out to spend time with your children the next day, but it gives you a feeling of joy and is a welcome reprieve from the demands of the world. The cookies that you indulge in cause you to feel bloated and depressed, yet while you are eating them you feel a deep sense of safety and security. That which you are seeking is not bad. What you desire is a state of happiness.

Your association with sweets—or certain foods like chips, bread, or french fries—, or alcohol, is one of strong pleasure:

joy, socializing, relief from emotional pain and comfort. These inner pictures of happiness around food and drink have been with you—and very likely your family—for a long time. However, you can dispel them and ultimately find the true happiness that you are searching for. In fact, you will discover that your food addiction and unproductive habits have prevented you from experiencing the very peace and joy that you seek. True happiness is connecting to the deep love buried inside yourself. By learning to love yourself and to care for your body, you will free yourself from the imprisonment of an endless food-craving cycle.

You will come to see that although sugar, like any drug, seems to be eliminating the undesirable states of emotional pain you experience in your life, it's actually keeping those very conditions you wish to move away from in place. Once you make that connection deeply on every level of your being—physically, emotionally, mentally and spiritually—something will click inside and you will naturally find yourself repulsed by or indifferent to sugary foods, and instead drawn toward those foods that nourish you.

Your perceptions of empty-calorie, processed, carbohydrate-rich foods will change, so that you are no longer attracted to the selections that are harmful to you. As you employ the methods that you will learn here, you'll notice that the more you select foods from the high-nutrition category—water-rich, whole, unprocessed foods with protein, healthy fat, and the least amount of complex carb to make your food taste good, in balance—the less hunger and craving you will experience. When we are eating the right amount of healthful foods that we enjoy, with occasional treats that will not reel us back into addictive behavior, we feel light and free. What a relief it is not to have to use stimulants just to get through the day.

No matter how long your self-sabotaging behaviors have been going on, you can learn to free yourself by changing your inner state naturally when you travel through the different parts of yourself to your source of strength. You'll learn to gain energy and vitality without needing to drug yourself with food. You will learn to become conscious of the triggers that cause you to overeat, eat in unhealthy ways, or reach for addictive substances and change your response to these triggers.

Relating to Food in a New Way

Before you can learn the tools that can update your unproductive responses to life, you need to commit to changing your entire way of relating to food. Food is not here to make you happy, or to distract you or comfort you. Food is here to sustain you—it is the fuel that makes your motor run. Without this realization, you are likely to continue to sabotage yourself. Yes, you always want to enjoy your food. In fact, that is one of the most important principles in this approach. However, enjoying food does not necessitate overindulging. In fact, you'll discover that in a way the less you eat—eating just enough to satisfy physical hunger only—the better you will feel. On the other hand, you do not want to experience too much hunger. Hunger is a sensation that can quickly lead you to overeat or choose unhealthy foods. You'll learn ways to eliminate hunger without eating too much food. You'll discover how power breathing, physical movement and even herbs like medical grade CBD, can help to regulate your blood sugar and eliminate excess hunger and cravings.

Why Certain Foods Make You Hungry

Often it's because of the types of foods you choose that you experience frequent physical hunger or feel insatiable. Refined white sugar and other sweeteners actually mask the body's natural signals of feeling full. This is why it is possible to consume so many calories when eating sugary foods. When the foods you eat are devoid of nutrients, your body continues to send out signals to the brain to eat more because it is still waiting for the nutrients it desperately requires to function in an optimum way. When we eat foods that are high in nutrients, the appetite naturally shuts off when we have eaten enough. However, when the foods and liquids we consume are high in sugar or caffeine, that natural system is bypassed—and we are often left feeling insatiable.

Typically, the endocrine and nervous systems cooperate to let us know how much to eat and when to eat. But when we introduce large amounts of refined sugar or sugar substitutes into our diet (and particularly when we've been eating that way for years), we throw those systems out of kilter. The increased appetite induced by sugar does not signal a need for more sugar, but a craving for nutrients and vitamins, minerals, omega-3, water and fiber. When we continue to ignore the communication of our body by stuffing it with even more sweet, sugary, or simple carbohydrate types of food—liquid or solid, we perpetuate a condition in which our endocrine glands and organs—the pituitary, pancreas, adrenal, and thyroid, as well as the nervous system, are overworked and thrown out of balance.

From Struggle to Solutions

Your food addiction and unproductive eating habits such as overeating, snacking, emotional eating, night eating and binging are rooted in physiological and emotional cravings. Once you fulfill the underlying need that is causing you to seek these harmful substances, you will no longer reach for them automatically.

We are always driven by our needs. As you begin to get in touch with and meet your needs, you can end addictive behavior for good. This includes your physical need for energy, rest, relaxation, health, and a sense of well-being and your deeper need to feel love, happiness, inner peace, purpose, and connection with something greater than yourself.

You may find yourself repeatedly engaging in certain behaviors around food without ever really understanding the cause. Perhaps you have an insatiable urge for chocolate every time you have conflict with your child, spouse, or boss, but never made the connection that when your world feels shaken up and you feel scared, chocolate is your oldest source of love and comfort. Perhaps it gives you a sense of peace, safety, or even confidence. Maybe when you are socializing with friends, you tend to overeat certain carbohydrate-rich foods such as pizza. You may associate the pizza with bonding with others, having fun, and enjoying life. Perhaps what you are really seeking is a sense of connection and companionship. Everyone has a different form of addiction and a different cause, so try the following exercise to begin to identify the root of your problem and see how food affects you.

. . . .

EXERCISE: DISCOVERING YOUR TRUE NEEDS

1. Take out a sheet of paper and write down a scenario in your life that is causing you to struggle with
   food or sweets addiction. Perhaps you find yourself
   bingeing when you are home alone at night, or finding excuses to eat candy bars regularly. Maybe your
   difficulty is eating large quantities of bread when
   you go out to dinner. Write down the scenario that
   is challenging for you and your response to it—for
   example, "I'm sitting in the restaurant feeling fam-
   ished, the bread comes and it smells so good. I tell
   myself I shouldn't eat it, but then I can't resist, so
   I eat three pieces," or "I come home from a long
   day at work, where my boss makes unreasonable
   demands on me, and I automatically reach for a can
   of soda and a bag of pretzels to soothe my frazzled
   emotions." As you recall the scenario, write down
   what you are feeling at the time. Bored? Exhausted?
   Anxious? Stressed?

2. Write down the positive result that the negative
   behavior gives you. This step assumes that you
   would not be repeating the harmful behavior if it
   didn't fill some need for you, no matter how much
   more in touch you are with the painful outcome it
   produces. Maybe raiding the refrigerator nightly
   helps you relax before bed and release some of the
   stress of the day's events. Perhaps the candy bars
   you reach for give you energy and help spur your
   creative juices when you are working on a project.
   The bread you consume may help you feel safe as

you sit down to dinner with friends or colleagues. Jot down any benefit you can think of to continuing with your unwanted habit.

3. Now write down how you feel afterward. After your evening eating spree you may feel sick, full, regretful, stuffed, and angry with yourself. Write these feelings down. Following the chocolate splurge you may find yourself depressed, hopeless, wired, aware of feeling uncomfortable in your clothes, or irritable. After you consume the bread, perhaps you feel bloated, uneasy, regretful, bad inside, and embarrassed, and perhaps even ravenously hungry.

4. How do you want to feel? This may seem obvious, but write it down. Embellish on the qualities that you wish to experience in your life, no matter how far from your current reality they appear to be. You may want to feel at peace, able to fall asleep easily at night without using food as a drug. Maybe you want to concentrate easily and feel creative and alive, having no need for harmful stimulants. It's likely that you wish to experience yourself as relaxed in social situations, happy, and feeling confident.

Now take a moment to assess what you have learned about yourself. Do you see how you are using certain foods—or categories of food—to fill your deeper needs? There is nothing intrinsically wrong with wanting to fill your needs, whether they be for love, safety, control, power, integrity, self-esteem, or peace. The issue is that continuing to try in vain to fill your needs with food, substance or alcohol keeps you in a state of feeling unfulfilled and in some level of emotional, or perhaps physical, pain. The way to freedom from this perpetual cycle of addictive behavior and its dire consequences is to become conscious of what's really happening inside you, but without judging yourself.

Filling Your Needs Directly

As you continue to read this book, keep in mind your own deeper needs. You will be learning new, productive ways to fill them. As you learn to fill your needs directly, you'll no longer reach for food as a way to numb unpleasant feelings. The methods outlined in *Easy Sugar Break-Up* will not only teach you a new, delightful way to eat and rid your body of physiological cravings for food, but it will also teach you to imagine a new way of being. By harnessing the power inherent in your imagination you can learn to use hypnotic techniques to change your life for the better.

Using Positive Imagery and Self-Hypnosis to Stop Cravings

Hypnosis is a state of relaxation, focused concentration, imagination, and heightened awareness. Whether we realize it or not, we use our imagination all day long, but often, unbeknownst to us, it is to our detriment. If you imagine that you are going to be late for your appointment and that your spouse will be angry with you, you create a physiological response in your body. It's likely that your stomach curls up into a knot, your jaw is clenched, and your breathing is shallow. When you run through mental movies of being fat the rest of your life and feeling too exhausted to get up off the couch when you come home from work, you implant these images into your very literal subconscious mind. Your subconscious mind does not evaluate whether these mental images are for your greater good—it simply follows orders, like a loyal servant.

The images you create in your mind have an effect on your body and on your impulses. In other words, if right now you take a moment to imagine the stress of sitting in traffic, using all your senses—imagining horns honking, the heat of the day beaming down on your windshield, and your mind racing with thoughts about getting to a very important meeting on time, you will realize that your body responds physiologically to the pictures you create in your mind. Now if you imagine that you are sitting at a red light, but that you are going to get together with a dear friend this evening—someone you can't wait to spend time with, or if you remember the tranquility of floating in the water on a beautiful, sunny day (in the shade, if you prefer), or resting in a hammock with a captivating book, the air fragrant with spring or fall, you will create a completely different reaction in your body. Most likely your blood pressure will go down, your muscles will relax, and your skin temperature in your fingers and toes will go up as your blood vessels relax and dilate as you let go. Perhaps you will even become aware of a relaxed smile coming to your lips or your favorite song floating on your tongue as you bask in images that make you feel good and alive. The images that play over and over in your mind are the ones that create how you feel, your physiological state (tense versus relaxed), and ultimately the behaviors you choose.

The behaviors you engage in—whether it's eating a fresh salad daily or heading straight for the Coke machine when you get to work—are based on the pictures you hold in your mind about yourself. These images create patterns of behavior that are like a traffic pattern on carpet, and just as predictable.

You can use this understanding entirely to your benefit. When you catch yourself imagining detrimental scenarios, such as your spouse bringing home Chinese food laced with sugar and MSG, and you feeling compelled to pig out on it, change the movie that's running through your mind. Affirm that you are in control. Instead, switch to an inner fantasy with you as the heroine, whipping up a delicious and healthy stir-fry, chock-full of fresh vegetables, free from additives and chemicals. Even if this exact scenario does not occur tonight, this week, or this month, know that your thoughts are creative, particularly the ones you repeat over and over with strong emotion. In fact, we often draw to ourselves that which we think about most, especially when our thoughts are coupled with strong images and emotions. This is what makes self-hypnosis and imagery so effective.

When you rehearse negative, hurtful scenarios, such as overeating at the wedding you are about to attend, and generate strong emotions in response to this fear, your worst-case scenario is far more likely to happen than if you imagined yourself instead truly enjoying the people you are with, drinking seltzer water with lime, eating the foods that you enjoy in moderation, and dancing to the upbeat music while fully engaged in the day's celebration.

In this book you will learn how to practice, in your mind, taking the actions that will lead you to your desired result. If you want to stop eating sugar, for example, you will imagine yourself instead enjoying and reaching for healthy snacks so that you are not hungry. Tune into your deeper need— the need for sweetness in your life—and imagine yourself filling that need in ways that satisfy you from the inside.

Turn yourself completely off to sugar or excessive alcohol consumption by playing and replaying the memories that exacerbate the pain associated with your sugar addiction. Make the images real for yourself by engaging all of your senses. In order to break long-standing habits, you will build momentum with the mental film clips you create of your new behaviors. Hypnosis is based on the use of imagery and suggestion as well as constant repetition to achieve a desired effect. You can use the principles of waking hypnosis to finally take control of your life and your eating behaviors, and you will learn how to do this in the chapters to come.

Motivation and Intention: Two Necessary Ingredients

In order to be successful in breaking free from strong sugar cravings and living a healthier life, it is essential that you make a deep commitment to yourself that this is truly what you want and that you want it for the right reasons. This means that even though a part of you may want to prove to yourself that you can lose weight or get compliments or look better than your best friend, it is important to see beyond the superficial desires of your limited, egoic, self. In other words, you may see a picture of an attractive, thin model and feel a stirring inside yourself say, "I really have to lose weight. I know I'll never look *that* good, but still the fat on my body is really disgusting." While this may provide some motivation for you, in the long run it probably won't get you very far. But if you can learn to travel deep inside your heart to the part of you that truly wishes to honor your body and to live a more purposeful life, that will be a greater incentive for you.

As you begin your journey deeper within, through the

methods you will learn, and relate more fully to your greater nature—your core—your reasons for wanting to eat in a healthy, balanced way will reflect that. When you are completely ready to be free from the painful limitation of a life controlled by addiction to sugar and simple carbohydrates and possibly weight obsessions, you are ready to set your deep intention to change and commit to the necessary follow-through. An intention is an inner quality of purpose that comes alive when you set a goal for yourself that you are committed to achieving.

Motivation is the greatest key to your success. I feel certain that the reason I was able to eliminate sugar from my diet successfully and consistently over these years is because I linked my actions of choosing healthy food and exercising in moderation to my greatest value: mental, physical, emotional and spiritual health. Once I saw the direct cause and effect between the foods and liquids I was consuming and the result they were having on my life—the fatigue, mood swings, PMS, anxiety, and the potential for heart disease and diabetes—I could not continue to justify eating in the old way, no matter how good the food tasted or how much pleasure I was receiving. I soon realized that the pleasure was an illusion, or certainly short-lived compared to the pain my lifestyle was causing me.

I could also see that the road I was traveling on was certain to lead to increased pain in the future. I began to consider the alternative to breaking free from food addiction—physical and mental illness and a compromised lifestyle—and felt the fear of choosing such an option. This healthy fear forced me to act in a way that was congruent with my deepest values. This is an example of learning from our legitimate fears. Sometimes our fears, as painful as they are, are warnings of what might actually happen if we continue to follow a particular course of action, and can therefore help to steer us in the direction that we truly want to go.

No matter how far we have traveled on a path that has not been for our greatest good, we always have the option of choosing again. This is one of the greatest blessings in life. And even though we may not have the same choices we did at a younger age, since we cannot undo the past, we can certainly make decisions today that will insure that we have a more desirable future than we would if we simply continued to relate to ourselves on the same autopilot—recycling the same thoughts, feelings, and actions that we always have. Does this take inner strength? It certainly does, but no matter how weak-willed you may perceive yourself to be, the strength is within you, and you can learn how to access it. The purpose of the tools I will share with you, including the Break-Your-Craving-State Technique, is for you to get in touch with and own the power that is—and always has been—within you, no matter how unaware you may have been of it. You may be oblivious to the beating of your heart, or even the fact that your lungs are breathing, and yet it is occurring every second. In the same way, there is a force within you that can not only free you from perpetuating unproductive habits, forever, but also propel your life and happiness to new heights, when you learn how to access it.

Making a Commitment to Yourself

Human desire is incredibly powerful, and when you set a strong intention for yourself you set into motion a chain of events that makes your goal achievable. This is quite different from sending wishes into space with no commitment on your part to engage in the behaviors that make your desire more likely to manifest. With a wish, there is a vague hope that something will happen to change your current set of circumstances, but no course of action is set in place to assure that it does. An intention, however, when set from the deepest part of you, has the potential to reconfigure your entire life. Setting an intention implies certainty, and you can feel this sense of assuredness in your body. Be certain about your ability to access your inner power and make permanent change. Being in control of your life and your eating habits, free from any substance addiction, truly is your birthright. All you have to do is claim it. You were not created to be obsessed with food, waiting for your next "fix" and having your entire life revolve around your next meal. You have the potential to be free, to be happy, and to connect to yourself and the people around you in a much more loving and profound way. Setting your intention to do so is your first step. Without an intention or commitment to a new way of life, there can be no result.

You would most likely get a different result if you set your intention from your limited conscious, analytical mind as opposed to coming from your heart and soul, where you hold a profound connection to your greater self—your deepest inner wisdom and source of creativity and love. Therefore it's important to learn how to travel beyond the mental chatter of the mind and access the deeper parts of your being. When you make your absolute commitment to change your life and you declare this inner resolve from your deep heart as opposed to your outer personality, you automatically gain the higher wisdom, strength, courage, and patience that your inner being carries to the task that lies ahead. You no longer have to do it all by yourself— meaning your small outward self. Now all the greater qualities that are inherently part of your higher nature become available to help you achieve your goal.

Why Your Core Values Hold the Key

When your intention is tied to your deepest values, you automatically get in touch with the motivation necessary to create the outcome you desire. For example, you may place a high value on your close relationships with friends. At some level, complaining about your issues with food or your weight may be a way of bonding with people you care about. However, when you understand that this form of connection is just keeping you stuck in old patterns and that your real value is friendship, you may choose to enlist your closest buddy as a workout companion instead. Now your bond becomes healthier and more productive, improving the quality of both of your lives.

If you are like me, freedom may be a top priority for you. So ask yourself, "What does freedom mean to me?" You may think freedom means "getting to eat whatever I want, whenever I want." However, upon further analysis, you are likely to realize that the outcome of living that way may very likely be compromised health or energy level or struggling with an overweight condition, and actually having less freedom because you become a slave to your own addiction. Therefore, if you truly wish to honor what you value—in this case freedom—you will set your intention to choose behaviors that, in fact, honor that.

Maybe you value truth as a virtue you wish to uphold in your life. Take a moment now to examine your life and notice if you are being truthful with yourself. You may tell yourself things like, "I can't keep myself from bingeing. I have no willpower." Are these statements true, or are they just limited beliefs based on old programming from the past? Set your intention to be honest with yourself. An honest intention may sound like this: "I set my intention to tell myself the truth.

That means that if I have an uncontrollable urge for frozen yogurt, I will be honest with myself about what I am feeling (perhaps weak and powerless), and I will be honest with myself about my deep desire to break free from the compulsions of the past and choose new behaviors. I acknowledge that even though I am not in touch with it, there is a greater strength within me that I am learning to access." When you are honest with yourself and honor your personal values, it becomes easier to make a new choice such as to do physical exercise, take a warm bath, or call a friend until the undesirable urge passes.

You can see why it is very helpful to know what your values are before setting your positive intention for your life, so that your intention can be guided by the values that are most important to you. In the following exercise you'll write down your most important values. A value is anything that you deem significant in the way you wish to live your life. You can use this list to help you: love, happiness, health, honesty, helping others, setting a positive example, truth, caring, patience, awareness, freedom, expression, challenge, beauty, creativity, serving God, intellectual pursuits, family, success.

. . . .

EXERCISE: CONNECTING WITH YOUR CORE VALUES

To elicit what you value most, ask yourself, "What is important to me in my life?" and write down what comes to you. Then when you have your list, compare and rate your various values by asking yourself, "Which of these do I value most, (for example, expression or setting a positive example)?" This will help you to develop a hierarchy of values. When you know what you value, you can begin to set an intention for yourself that is congruent with your deepest values. Using the list I have provided or coming up with your own, ask yourself what you value most for your life.

Setting Your Intention

In a few moments, you'll set your intention from the deepest part of yourself that you can access. From that place, you'll make a commitment to yourself to eliminate the substances that are controlling you and wreaking havoc on your life. At this point, please do not be concerned with obstacles such as certain situations you find yourself in that cause you to feel compelled to reach for addictive foods, physical withdrawal, or if part of you doesn't believe that fulfilling the intention you're about to set is possible for you. I want to assure you that the tools you'll be given in *Easy Sugar Break-Up* will help you with any challenges that may come up.

There is a great power in setting intention, and by contacting a greater force within yourself that is much more than your limited conscious awareness, you are setting the stage for a dramatic internal shift. What may not have been conceivable in the past can very likely become your new way of life. So take the risk—you have nothing to lose—and as best you can, open yourself on every level to something new and beautiful coming into your life. When you make your commitment to yourself, do it despite any reservations you may have about your ability to live up to what you are promising yourself.

In the next exercise, you'll begin to practice self-hypnosis by allowing yourself to drop into a light trance— behind your thoughts—and switching your focus from being outer directed to the innermost parts of your being. With daily practice, you'll learn to tap into the vast storehouse of power within and set new, positive outcomes for your life based on your true, deeper longings. Setting your intention will help you to solidify your inner commitment. It will also assist you in accessing your greatest strength and wisdom later when you learn the Break-Your-Craving-State Technique in Chapter 7. The tools given throughout this book are designed to make your self-hypnosis experiences more powerful and effective tools for achieving your goals.

During the exercise, I encourage you to just be with whatever you are experiencing—whether it be anxiety, fatigue, curiosity, or boredom—without trying to change or fix it. Just notice it as an observer. Trust that whatever is happening is occurring because it's supposed to. Just as the baby chick must struggle to break open the shell of the egg she is inhabiting to start her life in the world, it's important for you to understand that sometimes we also are in a state of struggle, and that there are no mistakes, regardless of our level of understanding at any particular time.

In a moment, put everything aside, shut your phone off, and make sure that you will not be disturbed. Then get in a comfortable sitting position and read through the following exercise once or twice. When you are ready, close your eyes and begin the exercise, "Setting Your Intention for Freedom from Sugar Addiction."

. . . .

EXERCISE: SETTING YOUR INTENTION FOR FREEDOM FROM SUGAR ADDICTION

Close your eyes, and begin by taking a few deep breaths. Just allow any cares of the day to slip away for now. You can return to them later. Focus on how your body feels as you sit comfortably. Let your belly, pelvis, and jaw become soft. Take your time. Feel your back and thighs against the chair and your feet on the floor. Be aware of your breath as it flows in and out. Now place your hand on your upper chest and breathe in and out underneath your hand. Focus on your breath flowing in and out under your hand. Begin to feel your personal connection to the outer world—the layer of your outer self, your personality—drop away

Notice any sensations, feelings, or images that may reside within you. Allow any thoughts that happen to come to you to drop from your mind into your heart. Imagine that your heart has arms or wings that can extend outward and envelope and hold your conscious, chattering mind.

Now allow yourself to sink even deeper into your heart. Imagine that you are going through a portal to a deeper layer of your being. Feel your breath going deeper into your chest and notice any feelings, textures, or even colors that may be in your awareness. Notice any sensations in your body as you let your consciousness scan your body from the top of your head down to the tips of your toes . . . Keep your hand on your upper chest to maintain the connection with your center. Imagine your breath flowing in and out underneath your hand. Imagine your breath pulling you deeper into your core and away from the outer world.

Using your breath to take you deeper still, keep your hand on your chest. Feel yourself going even deeper inside. Notice what you are aware of—perhaps a sense of expansion or a feeling of lightness. Enjoy the sensations and keep breathing deeply under your hand, into your deep heart. If you are experiencing any strong emotions, resist the urge to label or judge them and simply feel the power behind the feeling. Notice the aliveness of any sensation in your body, without any mental commentary about what it means. If your mind is racing, simply bow your head slightly to your heart to bring your focus down to your chest. Open your mouth slightly and relax your jaw. Making your breath slightly audible, like a loud sigh, may help you to sink deeper. You can also repeat a word or simple phrase, such as "deeper" or "one," that helps you to connect inside to your inner core. You may even see the word or phrase written in your heart in light—and feel yourself moving toward this light.

Now, as you continue to travel through your being to the subtle realms inside yourself, if you haven't already, begin to make contact with the greatest well of love that you can imagine—whatever that is for you. Use imagery to make this real for you. Envision a beautiful, fragrant rose, a delicate, exquisite orchid, a strong, powerful tree, or a vivid, awesome sunset to help you. Call upon any symbol that assists you in connecting with the highest light, goodness, or power that you can conceive of deep within yourself. Take the image you are using out of your mental field and bring it into your chest, deep within your heart. Imagine that source of goodness deep within you in whatever way is most real for you. Perhaps the image is that of yourself as a newborn baby, filled with love, trust, and spontaneity with yourself, your body, and others. Let yourself become full of the qualities that are inherent in your image. Spend a few moments basking in the feelings of great joy, peace, and freedom and just breathing them in. Feel the awe, and, if you like, bow even deeper to this presence of love and light deep within your own heart. Allow any thoughts to simply pass through, like clouds in the sky of your vast mind, as you open more and more to your image and to your connection to the higher qualities of love and safety in your core. Perhaps you may experience a surge of gratitude or unboundedness. If so, breathe it in. Bring the light all the way through your whole body, from the top of your head to the tips of your toes and beyond. To do this, you can imagine the image within your heart center expanding to include all of you.

From this deep place inside yourself, now—with a deep honoring of this presence of strength and wisdom that resides within you—set your intention to live your life healthy, free from sugar addiction, choosing to ingest only that which supports your greatest level of health and vitality. Remember the value that's most important to you and affirm to yourself that it's for this reason that you are determined to change your life for the better. Set your intention to be conscious of your thoughts and feelings and of everything that you put in your mouth. Set your intention to ask yourself, before you ingest anything, if this is what you are really wanting.

Imagine yourself keeping this commitment and what this would mean to you, both now and in the future. If thoughts of the past or voices of doubt about making such a promise to yourself creep in, command them to go and stay focused on the intense light in your heart and your deep bowing to your deeper self and the commitment that you are making to honor your body and your life from this time forward.

Set your own personal intention now. Feel the power of the promise you are making to yourself. Know that through your declaration, universal forces are being set in motion to help you to manifest this intention. Sit with that understanding and give thanks for the positive steps that you are taking to turn your life around and break your food addiction for good. Take whatever time you need, and then come back into the room when you are ready.

This is a very powerful exercise, and the more you do it, the greater the impact it will have on your life. When setting your intention, it is important to do it, not from your conscious mind, but from the deepest place within that you can access. Don't be discouraged if some days you are consumed with thoughts or doubt. That's perfectly natural. By doing this every day, you are beginning to create a new, positive habit. Also, the more you begin to see yourself in this new way, committed to honoring your body, the more natural this new image will become for you. These new thoughts about yourself will create new, positive eating and lifestyle behaviors that ultimately become your new healthy habits. Soon you'll find yourself naturally seeking healthier, more nutritious foods.

Realize that every time you connect with the deeper parts of yourself and the greater forces in nature—and set your intention based on that connection—you increase the probability that the intention you are setting in motion will come to fruition. Once you have tasted the deeper levels, it's natural to wish to reside in these hidden places of infinite beauty, safety, and spaciousness, where you can experience freedom from the limitations of your small self. The more you visit your true source of freedom within, the greater may be your desire to live from this place more and more. This sincere yearning is the motivation necessary to propel you forward as you begin to look at the blocks that are hindering your progress to freedom from food addiction and/or permanent weight loss and create a deeper, more profound connection to the treasures within you.

In later chapters, we will explore the obstacles found in the conscious and subconscious aspects of the mind and move toward the love you have for yourself in the deeper heart, beyond any conflict that may be currently present. You'll learn how to change your state from one of compulsive craving to that of inner peace and contentment.

Equally as important as addressing the emotional, psychological, and spiritual longings that lead to food, alcohol and stimulant cravings is looking at how the compulsion to eat simple carbohydrates and/or sweets is reinforced biologically when these foods or chemicals remain in your system. In the next chapter, we'll examine the real impact of sugar on your life and what perpetuates the endless physiological cravings for snack foods, alcohol, simple carbs, and sweets.

2. The Impact of Sugar on Your Life

Before we deal with the emotional side of eating, let's take a look at what's actually going on with your body when you binge or continually eat the wrong foods. The body is like a very delicate machine. It is very helpful to understand how the whole mechanism works and why we may feel so hungry again when we have eaten just a short time ago.

When you eat, your body begins to digest the food immediately with the enzymes that are secreted by the salivary glands in your mouth. When the carbohydrates you have eaten enter the blood, the pancreas is stimulated to produce insulin in order to lower the amount of sugar in the blood. This is a safety mechanism to prevent the sugar in the blood from rising too high. The sugar in the blood is then escorted by insulin into your body's cells to be used immediately or turned into glycogen to be stored in the liver and used later. Therefore, more insulin leads to stored glycogen and less blood sugar.

When the pancreas becomes over-stimulated as the result of an excessive amount of simple, refined carbohydrate and sugar being consumed over time, it can begin to overwork and send out too much insulin. The result is that the sugar in the blood is whisked away at a higher rate and stored as glycogen, resulting in low blood sugar. Basically, eating lots of processed carbs, chemically laden "food" and sugars causes blood sugar to lower, which affects how you feel, your cravings, and your health. When your blood sugar drops, the adrenal glands produce adrenaline, which signals the glycogen in the liver to be released, so you have sugar in your blood again. So even though you may have just consumed 2,000 calories, you feel ravenous, as well as jittery from the adrenaline.

The result is a state of blood sugar imbalance. This can induce cravings for more carbohydrates or create insatiable hunger as the body seeks to find equilibrium. Because the brain only uses glucose for fuel (as opposed to the other cells of the body, which can get their nourishment from protein and fat), often the symptoms we feel when our blood sugar is out of balance are dizziness, irritability, feeling faint, confusion, anxiety, worrying excessively, headaches, depression, exhaustion, mood swings, or indecisiveness. The brain is screaming for a "fix."

Unfortunately, if we respond to this plea with more processed carbohydrate and sugar-rich food, we are only feeding this vicious cycle and have little chance of getting off the roller-coaster of insatiable food craving. Consuming these foods perpetually keeps us in a state of wanting more. They truly are addictive!

Our only hope is to nip this painful situation in the bud by stabilizing the blood sugar to avoid the ups and downs. When we eat in a balanced way, selecting foods from the complex carbohydrate, protein, and healthy fat categories, making sure to eat water-rich, unprocessed foods with a high fiber content as much as possible, ingesting only small portions at a time, the insulin response from the pancreas is not so erratic, and sugar levels in the blood remain steady, thereby making us feel calmer and more satisfied. Also the adrenals calm down and we don't have that frantic feeling of being in an emergency situation, often accompanied by a blood sugar reaction.

What Are Complex Carbohydrates?

A carbohydrate is considered to be either simple or complex depending on how many molecules it consists of. Because simple carbohydrates—such as sugar in all its forms and white flour products—have fewer molecules, they require minimal digestion and are absorbed into the bloodstream very quickly. The rapid rate at which sugar enters the blood actually makes it like a drug. Refined sugar—which if you read labels is in almost all processed foods—floods the body and causes a stress reaction.

Complex carbohydrates, on the other hand, are starches such as those in whole-grains, potatoes, and legumes that are made up of three or more sugar molecules. When we eat complex carbohydrates, it takes the digestive system more time to break them down into sugar. When they are combined with protein and healthy fat, complex carbohydrates provide the body with a slow, steady supply of sugar rather than an abrupt onslaught, and our health improves.

All foods ultimately turn into glucose in the body. The glucose or sugar is what provides us with the energy we need so that all our bodily systems can function properly. However, when we eat sugar or simple carbohydrates, the glucose is released into the bloodstream immediately, and unfortunately this causes harmful side effects. It is far better to have the fuel that our bodies need come from foods that are whole rather than refined.

The process of refining sugar or flour is accomplished by extracting the active ingredient from the plant rather than maintaining the plant in its natural state. For example, a whole food would be grains of wheat, rye, or barley with the husk intact as opposed to white flour where the bran has been removed. When whole-grains are refined, they are left devoid of nutrients, and fiber, which slows down the rate of digestion and absorption, is not available to the body. Why does the food industry perpetually strip the husk from grains and add refined sugar to most food products? Because it preserves the shelf life. The important thing to consider, however, is the effect on your body and your quality of life once you become consumed with cravings.

Eating to Keep Blood Sugar Levels Steady

To have a stable blood sugar level and be free from food cravings and obsessions, you will need to eat in a way that creates balance inside your body. When you are in a state of equilibrium, you will feel satisfied with the foods you eat, and you will eat as a way to satisfy physical hunger and keep your blood sugar stabilized rather than simply due to appetite.

Be assured that you will still fully enjoy the foods you select, but will be much more connected to what type of food your body needs in the moment, based on what you have already eaten. In other words, if you had a complex carbohydrate such as a sweet potato at the last meal—though it is a healthful choice—you will begin to intrinsically have a sense that the next thing you eat needs to balance that so that you don't end up with too much carbohydrate in your system. That's because even complex carbs, in excess, can affect your blood sugar level. You need to keep your blood sugar steady by including high-quality protein (for many of us, this has to be animal protein to cure the cravings), omega-3 healthy fat such as extra virgin olive oil or flax seed oil, water-rich food such as vegetables, and complex carbohydrate, in your meals. Because you just ate a carb—albeit a complex one—a good way to restore and maintain an inner stability would be to choose protein, healthy fat, and green vegetables, such as a salad with extra virgin olive oil dressing and broiled salmon on top. When we are in a healthy and balanced state, after we eat carbohydrate or protein, we tend to crave water-rich food such as veggies. The body always seeks equilibrium. However, when we are out of balance, we just keep craving more carbs in a thwarted attempt to self-correct. The more simple, processed, refined carbs we eat, the more out-of-balance we become.

Eating vegetables at every meal also assures that your body is ingesting plenty of fiber, which is essential for optimal health and digestion, as well as providing a feeling of fullness. (Fruit—both fresh and dried—is high in fiber as well, but because of its high sugar content may not be the best choice for many people, as fruit can increase cravings for more sweet foods.) Fiber slows the rate at which sugar and fat enter the bloodstream, which lowers your potential for food cravings or weight gain.

When the blood sugar is steady, you are in a state of flow—open to life and feeling fully alive. In this state, cravings subside, and you have a new freedom to enjoy food, but no longer be obsessed with it. What keeps you in this steady state is eating in a balanced way, selecting items from all the healthful categories of food, drinking lots of water to keep your body clean and well-hydrated, eating lots of fiber-rich foods to slow the rate at which the food is turned to sugar in the body, exercising to increase metabolism, and eliminating all those harmful, processed, high-sugar, high–trans fat foods from your system.

As long as sugar is in your system, you are very likely to continue to crave it, particularly if you are sensitive to it. It is very important to be aware of the many hidden sources of sugar. If you are going to eat processed food (and it's difficult to avoid completely), read the labels. Other words for sugar are honey, maple syrup, glucose, lactose, fructose, maltose (anything that ends in -*ose*), sorbitol, alcohol (such as white wine), and corn syrup. Even sugar substitutes can cause the same blood sugar reaction that refined sugar does. When it comes to determining which foods are best for you and which foods need to be avoided, there is no exact science. It is much more of an art to learn to know your body and be aware of its predictable reactions. Realize that the more processed the foods you are eating, the more difficult it may be to keep your blood sugar steady and avoid cravings.

Recently I was on a cruise ship and noticed that after a couple of days I started to eat foods that I typically don't eat at home. Sure, I was avoiding all the desserts, since they are not an option for me, but I started to eat more bread and butter than I was used to, and certainly larger quantities of food. Interestingly, I noticed that by eating more and choosing foods that were not best for my system, I actually began to feel hungrier and much less satisfied with food than I am used to. Also, I noticed that because there was such a large assortment of different foods, I was eating more than I normally would. Studies show that the greater the variety of food that is available, the more people will eat. That finding confirms for me my decision to simplify my usual diet (eating style) by eating simple, basic foods most of the time. For me, this actually makes my life easier and makes it easy to stick with a sensible food plan. Chapter 8, "High-Nutrition Eating," will help you, too, to come up with a food plan that works for you, without ever feeling like you are deprived or on a diet. You'll learn how you can keep your body fed with just enough delicious, nutritious food to ward off any sense of physical hunger.

How Do Certain Foods Affect You?

As you notice your own personal patterns around food, you will be better able to discern the effect of various foods on your blood sugar, and how they take you out of a state of flow. If you use an outside source (like a certain diet) to tell you what to eat, you run the risk of feeling deprived because you haven't internalized the desire to choose certain foods, and instead are following directions to get a certain result. Also, the advice you are given may not be entirely true for you personally.

For example, you may read about using the glycemic index or glycemic load to measure the rate at which a food turns to glucose in the blood. This system can be very helpful, however, realize that the findings are not hard and fast. For example, according to this index, a white potato may be scaled higher than ice cream (meaning ice cream would cause less of a blood sugar response than a potato). This may be true for some people, but I would highly recommend that you question concepts like this to determine what's true for yourself. For me, I enjoy a small potato every so often, with sea salt and a little butter or cheddar cheese. I eat it with the skin to get all the vitamins, minerals, and fiber. When I add a small steak and a large green salad to my meal, I feel completely satisfied, and my blood sugar remains stable. This meal keeps me in a balanced state.

Ice cream, on the other hand, is not anything I would consider eating at this stage in my life. I feel like it would set me back into severe food cravings, and the momentary pleasure of a good taste is simply not worth it. I intuitively know this, so it doesn't matter if there's a chart that tells me that ice cream is a better choice for blood sugar than a potato. It just doesn't ring true for me. I encourage you to also learn to trust yourself around food. Diets like Paleo, Weight Watchers, Raw, Vegan or any of the other myriad of diets out there, may have merit. But as long as you are following someone else's eating plan, you may not be being true to your own body's unique needs. Notice your reactions and honor them. It takes practice to find the foods that keep your blood sugar stable. The more you select healthy, water-rich, whole, unprocessed foods the more you will begin to crave those foods. For most people with sugar addiction, animal protein eaten at regular intervals throughout the day is the major secret to keeping the blood sugar steady and warding off hunger. All types of fish, lamb, beef, turkey, duck, and chicken are the best sources. Including some dairy is fine, however, I do not recommend eating yogurt or drinking milk as a substitute for meat, poultry, or fish, since milk and yogurt actually contain more carbohydrate than protein. Also, when consuming dairy, notice your reaction to the sugar in milk products, not only regarding digestion, but the effect of the dairy products on your entire system. There has been evidence that for some people, milk and yogurt (and of course ice cream) can trigger hunger or cause fatigue and other blood sugar–related symptoms.

A Word About Animal Protein

Eating meat nowadays has become very controversial. To admit you eat meat is actually very bold, and in many social circles, is not politically correct at all. It's not unusual for me to get angry Facebook comments and posts from vegans and animal right activists. Believe me, I get it! I understand the environmental, social and economic issues surrounding meat consumption. Concerns about how inhumanely animals are treated, or the health risks of eating too much saturated fat, are absolutely valid. Still I believe it's so important to be authentic and talk about the true reasons why for some of us, meat is an essential staple for health and balance. The reason I eat meat and encourage other people who have a pre-diabetic or a "carb-sugar addict gene" to do the same, is because there is no other food that can balance blood sugar as well as meat does. One of my clients who came to me for a private hypnosis session once said to me, "Meat is my medicine." I thought that was brilliant. That statement sums up for me why meat is such a necessary stable in my "diet." I put that word in quotes because I am not on a diet, nor do I advocate any particular diet. My goal is to help you find and stick to a sensible eating style for life. For me, without including meat in my daily food intake, I would be grossly overweight and unhealthy. Eating meat allows me to stay in balance and eat much less food in general. Allow me to clarify. I'm not talking about devouring huge, greasy, steaks on a regular basis. My animal protein intake is comprised of eating hormone free, anti-biotic free meat, in very small portions, always balanced by large amounts of water rich, plant food, such as salad and vegetables, with small amounts of complex carbs, and enough healthy fat. As much as I would love to be a vegetarian—in fact I am a vegan wanna-be—including meat in my eating plan—allows me to maintain an inner state of balance—which is the physical key to freedom from all addiction.

Enjoy Your Food!

The secret to success is making sure that the foods you select taste good to you. Don't deprive yourself. It is much more satisfying to have a small amount of a food that you really love (as long as it won't cause an upset with your blood sugar) than to try to satisfy yourself with foods that you don't enjoy at all.

For example, though I will never eat ice cream again, once in a while I will indulge in a few corn chips. I'd rather eat just a handful of salted and oiled chips than a whole bag of fat-free, salt-free chips. Neither choice is particularly healthful. But the salted chips will satisfy me whereas the fat-free, salt-free variety will just keep me in a state of deprivation and overeating. To make the chips a better choice, I select the ones from the health food store, which are made with healthier oils, added sesame seeds (which are high in calcium), and sea salt rather than table salt. An even better choice would be fat-free lavash or wraps—heating them in the oven until they are crisp and breaking them into small, chip-size pieces. Then if I add delicious avocado (healthy fat) and some meat (preferably organic and hormone-free) and cheese (just enough to make it taste good) to the chips, I am likely to be quite satisfied for several hours. So if ten minutes later the ice-cream truck comes ringing its bell on my street, I won't even notice it. But a bag of stale, tasteless, or low-calorie chips eaten alone or with low-calorie salsa would definitely send me wanting something else. That's why the trick is learning to understand your body's blood sugar mechanism and working with it. It's not about suffering!

Some people think that when they give up ice cream, they'll start eating yogurt or frozen yogurt, or even worse, fat-free yogurt. Beware of anything labeled "fat-free." Usually that just means "added sugar or sweetener." What you give up in fat, you gain in sugar or sugar substitutes, and when it comes to maintaining a normal blood sugar level and a healthy weight, the price you pay for eating sugar is much higher. For many people yogurt (even plain yogurt) may stimulate cravings as much as ice cream does. It may or may not be the case for you, but please be aware of it as a possibility.

Your Body Needs All Types of Foods

However, please don't think of carbohydrates as being "bad" or go on a carbohydrate-free diet. Again, I want to emphasize that we need food from all categories in our diet.

The proteins we eat are broken down into amino acids that become the basic building blocks for all the body's cells, hormones, and neurotransmitters. Even though protein can be turned into glucose in the absence of carbohydrate, it is preferable to fill the body's requirement for glucose by eating carbs, so that the protein can be reserved to fill the vital function of building our cells.

Carbohydrates are necessary. They help to increase our brain's supply of the feel-good chemical serotonin, which produces a calming, anxiety-reducing effect. Often reaching for chocolate, pie, pizza, or chips is a way to self-medicate and fill the body's need for serotonin. The drawback to this approach is the ensuing weight gain and the painful cycle of sugar addiction that occurs as a result. When we eat complex carbohydrates, which, again, are carbs in their natural state, with the husk from the grain intact, as part of a balanced diet, we fulfill the body's need for serotonin, but without the negative side effect of constant craving. This occurs because the carbohydrates we eat increase the amount of an amino acid called tryptophan's ability to reach the brain.

When we eat carbohydrates and insulin is secreted, the blood sugar is lowered and competing amino acid levels are reduced, thereby giving tryptophan the ability to cross the blood-brain barrier and increase the level of the feel-good chemical serotonin. Tryptophan, which comes from protein, is the necessary precursor to serotonin. Therefore eating protein and complex carbohydrate together insures that adequate amounts of serotonin are produced in the brain without stimulating the adrenals and pancreas to produce high levels of energy-depleting hormones.

The more you get in touch with how your body feels, the easier it is to let physical hunger determine what and when you are going to eat. If you have a dieting mentality and are already in a state of deprivation, it's much harder to turn away from the abundance of sweets that you are probably surrounded by as you go through your daily life. However, if you know what your dietary limitations are and accept them fully, you can begin to fill your daily meals with foods that truly satisfy you and that don't set you up for addictive, compulsive behavior. The items you choose may certainly include a variety of tastes, textures, and flavors that you thoroughly enjoy. When you eat this way regularly, then when you encounter a situation where a food is being served that is not an option for you, it isn't nearly the big deal it would be if you were already coming from a place of extreme hunger, deprivation, or not having your needs met.

Success Secret

I had a client recently who sheepishly admitted to me, "I just don't like vegetables. Can you hypnotize me to like vegetables?" she asked. Before we did any hypnosis, I wanted to help her to get in touch with her own inner power to make smart choices. I asked her, "How do you prepare your vegetables?" She explained to me that growing up, the only vegetables she saw were those in a can. Lara then guiltily explained that she tries to steam vegetables the way she has been told to, but she just doesn't like how they taste. I assured Lara that even the healthiest eaters would likely agree with her. Eating healthfully does not mean eating foods that taste like cardboard or sawdust. Food needs flavor. Over-cooking any food, including fresh vegetables, is likely to ruin it. Your healthy food has to taste good if you want to re-train your brain to like it (especially when it's competing with the kind of chemical concoctions the food industry is spending millions of dollars creating, to be sure to hook your taste buds, with decadent combinations of sugar, sugar substitutes, salt, coloring, additives, etc.).

There are so many delicious ways to prepare vegetables: grilling, broiling, stir frying, sautéing. Combined with the least amount of healthy fat, like extra virgin olive oil, perhaps mixed with tahini (sesame paste) and miso (fermented soy paste to give it a little healthy salty flavor), veggies of all types can be a culinary delight. Also combinations make a huge difference. At night if I am hungry, I may take a small amount of anti-biotic free, 85% lean ground beef, sprinkled with tasty sea salt, high in potassium, and cook it up with some organic cabbage or brussel sprouts. I choose meat that isn't totally lean because taste is such an important factor for long term success. It's highly unlikely to ever over-eat plain meat, but if it doesn't taste good, it will leave me wanting something else. Because it's rich and tasty, with some natural fat, and I am not adding any kind of chemical sauce, it's easy to just have a tablespoon or two of the meat, with a big heaping portion of cabbage cooked up with the protein, and be completely satisfied.

A delicious way to cook up zucchini, eggplant or yellow squash is simply to cut it into long slices, place on a slightly oiled baking sheet, and broil for about 8 minutes, until it's crisp. If you are committed to never dieting again and living your life at your perfect ideal weight, it's essential that you prepare all your food so it tastes delicious and satisfying.

Another delicious option that can work any time of day is an omelet, cooked in olive oil, and loaded with spinach, leeks, and other tasty vegetables.

Your Personal Food Map

It's helpful to think of your dietary selections as following a continuum. Draw an imaginary line, either on paper or in your mind's eye. On one end, think of the foods that you know are harmful to you—the ones that seem to set off compulsive eating for you. On the other end of the spectrum, list the foods that are the most healthful ones for you—the foods that make you feel light, healthy, and energetic. Then, in the middle, write down or think of the foods that are neutral, or the items that generally don't cause the pendulum to swing in either direction.

So, for example, if I were to draw such a map for myself, at the far left side would be the foods that are likely to lead me to illness, obesity, compulsive eating, or disease—since I feel a strong potential within myself for a serious blood sugar disorder. These foods at the far left would be any highly processed food, particularly with a high level of simple, refined carbohydrate. This would include macaroni and cheese; ice cream; store-bought cookies or cake; foods prepared with sugar, molasses, or honey; candy or chocolate; Cheetos, potato chips, and other similar processed snack foods; milk-based soups; and rich, creamy, or chemically laden sauces.

Then on the far right would be the foods that are best for me: fresh green salad; green, purple, or yellow vegetables including leeks, collards, kale, cabbage, zucchini, eggplant, and broccoli. Also at the far right are healthy fats: extra virgin olive oil, flaxseed oil, and grape seed oil. Equally as healthy for me is animal protein: eggs, chicken, turkey, lamb, tuna, salmon (or any fish), and beef, preferably without hormones or antibiotics. All processed meats such as sausage, hot dogs, bacon, or lunchmeats would go over to the left-hand category, as they are filled with sweeteners, in addition to other harmful chemicals.

In the middle, but closer to the right side, are delicious toppings that I can eat in moderation such as avocado, cheese, almond butter and dry roasted, unsalted nuts.

Remember, this is my map. Yours may be a little different. Each of us needs to discover which foods are best for us and which foods we need to cut back on or avoid. Interestingly, there are many "healthy" foods that I also need to be careful with and place in the middle category. These are all the delicious root vegetables: potatoes, sweet potatoes, butternut squash, and whole-grains such as brown rice, whole-grain pasta, and oatmeal. I do eat them fairly regularly, but always eat them in combination with greens and vegetables, fat, and/or protein to keep my system in balance.

The foods on the far left are foods I have learned, over time, that I need to stay away from. However, along the middle (a little closer to the left) are many foods that I also need to be careful with, but that I consider a treat and can get away with once in a while, as long as I am careful to always bring myself back to a balanced state. The middle—toward the left— foods include bread products and foods made from them, as well as fruit. So if I want to eat bread (or any wheat or corn product such as pizza, bagels, or nachos) once in a while, I do, but I am very aware that if I cross a certain threshold, I will begin to crave these foods more and more, and interestingly, healthy food may not look as appealing to me anymore. It's very helpful to have the recognition that when our bodies are filled with processed, refined, high-sugar foods, we perpetuate cravings for these foods and increase the likelihood of becoming turned off to healthy foods such as vegetables and salad. Because for me, bread products are in the middle of my dietary continuum, I can eat them in moderation, meaning once in awhile, without setting off a binge.

I do want to emphasize, however, that I do not have the same luxury with the foods on the far left. I stay away from them the way an alcoholic avoids liquor, simply because I know from past experience that these foods would set me up for a very painful binge or create a painful mental obsession with sweets. On the other hand, by not depriving myself totally and eating very tasty foods from the middle category, while making the majority of my selections from the category on the far right, I get to enjoy scrumptious food every day. Also, by incorporating enough healthy fat in combination with more water-rich foods, I get the benefit of excellent taste sensations. I also use condiments such as sea salt or low-sodium, alcohol-free soy sauce and herbs to flavor my foods, making them delicious.

When we deprive ourselves—for example by going on a carbohydrate-free diet—even though we can get tremendous health benefits by balancing the blood sugar and losing weight over the short run, we are probably going to end up in a very serious binge over the long run. Remember, the body needs carbohydrates, along with protein, salad/veggies and healthy fat, because it needs balance. What the body does not need is chemical processing. Our health depends on selecting all our foods in as close to their natural state as possible.

Compare your eating regime to balancing on a teeter-totter. Once you find the balanced approach that works for you, it's possible to eliminate cravings forever. The map I have described can be an extremely helpful way of doing this. If you balance your food choices on a daily or weekly basis, then you can finally stop having weeks or months where you are being "good" and avoiding all fattening (and tasty) food, only to experience the very painful swing of the pendulum, when you eat everything you want with wild abandon, causing serious consequences for yourself, in addition to strongly hurting your self-esteem.

Being Guided by Your Eating Behavior Pendulum

When you think of your dietary habits as following this continuum, it will be so much easier to nip compulsive eating in the bud, take control of your eating behavior pendulum, and swing it back in the direction of your conscious choice. For example, if you realize that you just stopped at McDonalds, and before you were even aware of what you were doing, you finished your daughter's Big Mac and fries, remind yourself that having these foods in your system is very likely (aside from making you feel bad physically or mentally) going to create a desire for more processed food as soon as these digest a little.

So be prepared. When the craving comes later in the day (or soon after) for an ice-cream cone (now that you've "blown your diet"), do not follow that impulse. Rather, look at your map and acknowledge to yourself that due to your mistake, you are now on the far left of your continuum, and make a choice to start eating foods on the right side of your chart when you are hungry again. Have celery or carrots on hand, or a spring mix salad with olive oil dressing.

Resist the urge to think of this as a punishment that you'll want to rebel against, and consider it a choice to keep you in a balanced, healthy state. The more you think about your dietary selections this way, the less little slipups like the fast food will matter. Also, ironically, you will be less likely to make them, because compared to the delicious and healthy food that becomes part of your regular regime, the greasy choices of the past begin to look repulsive. If this seems unlikely to you right now, realize that perhaps you have never truly allowed yourself to indulge in healthy food that is prepared with an adequate amount of healthy fat and flavor. Perhaps you equate healthy food with bland diet food.

On the other hand, some of my clients tell me that they love healthy food, and that this isn't the problem. They tell me that they just eat too much healthy food, or after they eat the delicious grains and vegetables or meat, they still crave sweets. Perhaps this may be the case for you, too. Too much of any kind of food can be toxic to the system. If you find that you are overeating even healthy foods, take time to write down the foods you are eating and look for patterns. There may be a certain flavor or item that sets off a tendency for you to binge. For some people that may be soy, dairy, eggs, or wheat. It's well worth your time to look for the culprit. Simplifying your diet by eliminating some of these common offenders can be a very effective way to naturally begin eating and desiring less food.

It can also be very helpful to eat more slowly and drink a full glass of water before each meal. If that is challenging for you, try experimenting with different types of water. I found that when I switched to distilled water, I could drink a lot more. I also created Slender Cider™ as a way to help myself and others drink more water, gently cleanse and stay alkalized (you'll learn more about how important alkalinity is for health, in chapters 8 and 11). Slender Cider is a liquid herbal concentrate of 11 therapeutic herbs in a base of organic, raw, apple cider vinegar, that you add to water. Sipping on Slender Cider in this way throughout the day, helps to physically eliminate cravings for salty and sweet foods. People have also used Slender Cider to kill cravings for alcohol and cigarettes, very successfully.

The Key to Health

One of the biggest obstacles to success I see over and over in my clients is black or white thinking. Either I am being "good" or "bad," "on a diet" or "off the diet." It can be much more productive to think in terms of, "Are my choices leading me closer to or further from my goal?" Let go of the judgment and criticism. Think of it this way: If you were driving from New York to Los Angeles and saw signs for Canada, would you keep going? Would you tell yourself, "Well, I've already been driving for 8 hours, so I might as well just stay on this road?" Of course, not! You would turn around as soon as you realized that you had made a mistake. In the same way, it's not about being perfect. If you suddenly realize that you just ate two "forbidden" cookies, why tell yourself, "I might as well just eat the whole box?" Every moment gives you an opportunity to make a new choice. And again, it's not necessary to be perfect or even "good." It's those judgments that hold you back from achieving success. Instead, imagine that all your choices are either bringing you closer or further from your goal, in each and every moment.

You have got to realize that your dream of being free from insatiable food cravings and compulsion around food is absolutely possible for you. Look around you. Yes, there are a lot of obese people to be found, and yet there are also millions of people who have learned how to have a healthy relationship with food. You can, too! The important thing is to know yourself and be honest with yourself.

If there are certain foods, or certain categories of foods, that cause you to become ravenously hungry (whether it's head hunger or stomach hunger), then these are foods that you will most likely need to avoid, at least for a period of time. I define head hunger as a headache, light-headedness, dizziness, confusion, or in some cases a strong, unwarranted emotional reaction. On the other hand, stomach hunger is when your belly is empty—perhaps growling. In either case, these types of foods may need to be avoided. Rather than seeing the need to abstain as a huge injustice and source of discomfort, you can turn that around to be a blessing for you. Just having the understanding and knowledge of yourself gives you the key to health and possible longevity.

Realize that it is absolutely possible to change your own biochemistry by modifying your dietary choices. Altering your biochemistry is one way to change your state on a physiological level. But why did your physical body get out of whack in the first place? It could be partly genetics, environment, and lifestyle over time that have caused you to engage in and perpetuate eating behaviors that have been destructive to you.

However, there is another reason, besides simply the unproductive eating habits you have developed over many years or the sweet taste of all the simple carbohydrate foods you've come to look forward to eating, why you are maintaining a lifestyle and eating habits that are impacting the quality of your life in a very negative way. Eating in an unhealthy or compulsive way, or not exercising, fills a need for you. Once we find new ways to fill the very real needs that we all have—such as finding peace and love within ourselves—and change our internal state from feeling overwhelmed or sad to feeling happy and contented, we can put an end to any destructive relationship with food we may have had in the past.

Part 2. Harnessing Your Inner Power for Success

3. Learning to Love Yourself

In order to free yourself permanently from the constant nagging of incessant food cravings by eliminating the foods that are responsible, it is imperative that you learn to love yourself fully. That doesn't mean denying the areas of your life that you would like to improve, but rather completely accepting yourself as you are and forgiving yourself for past mistakes. If you are like many of my clients who suffer from insatiable food cravings, you may be hard on yourself because you have an unrealistic image of perfection that you are trying in vain to live up to. Because that image is unrealistic and unattainable, you may often find yourself giving up and swinging to the other extreme, where you engage in behaviors that you know are harmful and counterproductive to what you wish to achieve.

You may think that if you had more willpower you would be able to eliminate unhealthy, fattening, empty-calorie foods from your diet. However, the secret is not having more willpower, it is increasing your belief that you are worthy to be free from food addiction and old, unproductive habits, and that this goal is attainable. You have willpower—think about the many other areas in your life where you display willpower. Often, at my seminars, when I ask the participants to think of their own personal obstacles to achieving their goals, someone will say that he or she is weak-willed.

When I question participants further about this, they smile when they realize that their loved ones often say the opposite about them: that they are in fact stubborn and strong-willed. When pressed, most people who initially say they have no willpower discover that they are displaying willpower in many other areas of their lives. What is even stronger in us than willpower is habit—specifically, unproductive eating habits that have developed over time. These habits include over-eating, binge-eating, night eating, eating when we are not physically hungry and emotional eating.

Most of us learned the habit of emotional eating when we made the connection as small children that ice cream or a lollipop made us feel better when we got hurt and helped us to quickly forget about our boo-boos. And even though, as an adult, you know that if you eat as a way to cope with any challenge in your life—whether it be depression, frustration, or boredom—the initial problem is only going to get worse; the subconscious program that tells you to eat so you'll feel better is controlling your life. The solution is to install a new, updated program.

If you feel that it is difficult to truly love and accept yourself, you may be overly identified with and judging your unproductive behaviors from the past. Who you are is not your thoughts or your behavior. How you feel about yourself is determined by what aspect of yourself you are focused on. The following exercise will help you to discover and focus on the strengths within you.

. . . .

EXERCISE: TAKING AN INNER INVENTORY

Take out a sheet of paper and make a list of the qualities that you love about yourself—those attributes that you would consider your assets, and also write down the evidence that you have. Then make a second list of what you would consider your liabilities. Now go through your list of liabilities and find exceptions to every item on the list.

For example, perhaps your list may look like this:

ASSETS	
Quality	*Evidence*
Caring	I listen to my children.
Generous	I help my sister financially.
Talented	I cook delicious meals for my family.
Giving	I volunteer at the local animal shelter.
Smart	I figured out how to stop the leaky faucet.
LIABILITIES	
Quality	*Evidence*
No control	I overeat constantly.
Impatient	I reacted so irritably when I had to wait.
Judgmental	I was really put off by my brother.
Ungrateful	I didn't want the scarf my mother gave me.

Now look at the evidence that you wrote down for your liabilities and find exceptions to the statements you made. So in the preceding example, under "no control," find an example of a time when you exercised control, for example maybe you stopped to help at a car accident and calmed down a hysterical woman, or you patiently helped your child to understand a difficult math assignment.

The purpose of doing this exercise is to learn that we all have every quality. We tend to think in black or white. Either I am a patient person or an impatient person. But the truth is that each of us is a complex combination of all personality traits, even though we may exhibit and identify with some more than others. If you believe your self-esteem is low, notice which attributes you identify within yourself. If you call yourself stupid, for example, be aware of how you aren't paying attention to the many talents that you do have or the areas in your life where you exhibit intelligence. Though you may have difficulty understanding how your computer works, you may be a whiz at keeping your plants thriving. Make a commitment to yourself to begin to take note of the areas in life where you do excel.

Acknowledge Your Successes

Rather than beating yourself up because you eat a loaf of bread every three days, praise yourself for having the discipline to work out a couple of times a week. I am not suggesting that you pretend areas of yourself and your life that are in need of improvement don't exist. I am, however, asserting that by giving yourself acknowledgement for your positive attributes and behaviors, you will increase the likelihood that they will continue and even spread to other areas of your life.

By recognizing and rewarding your successes you will begin to identify yourself as a person who can and does achieve the goals that you set for yourself.

Do you project your more noble qualities onto other people? For instance, you may admire a friend because she is so calm, even when she has to care for so many people. You may criticize yourself as too hurried to really enjoy the people who come to visit you. What you may be blocking out is that your friend has full-time help and doesn't work outside the home, whereas you may have a very demanding business that requires a great deal of your time and energy, and you may currently have little outside help.

By noticing that you are calm and caring, you can set your intention to be calmer and more caring with yourself when you are in situations that are particularly stressful. When you acknowledge your own self-discipline, instead of concerning yourself with how you are going to find time to work out at the gym, you may decide to get a stroller with hand brakes and Rollerblade with your babies, as an alternative. In other words, by focusing your energy on solutions, instead of on berating yourself, you can tap into your inner wisdom and find creative ways to achieve your goals, even with your life circumstance as it is.

Making New Connections

Understand that your compulsion around food is not an indication that you are a weak or undisciplined person. It simply means that in this area of your life, your behavior does not match your desire to be healthy and experience a deeper level of happiness. This could easily be the result of unproductive programming that's been going on for many years, coupled with a lack of understanding about the drug-like nature of certain foods and how choosing a diet of healthy, nutritious foods can free you from this painful cycle of insatiable food cravings.

These are not concepts that most of us have been taught as children. We often are not aware that a large reason we crave the foods we do and are turned off to other foods, is simply because our body craves/desires the foods we typically put into it. If I hadn't gotten sick at a young age, I probably would never have made the decision to stop drinking alcohol or eating sweet or processed, chemical-filled foods for good. So each of us in our own time becomes educated about what we have to do to achieve and maintain a higher level of health. It really is about making connections and then basing our decisions on the outcome of our discoveries. When I realize that if I overeat, I become lethargic or short-tempered, I now have the information necessary to make a new choice. Then, if I also become aware that when I select more water-rich foods, I have more energy, feel lighter, and am more likely to exercise and feel happier, it's easier to make the necessary changes in my lifestyle to insure that these behaviors happen more naturally and consistently.

The other empowering connection to make is that the more you eat healthy food, the more you crave/desire the same, thus insuring freedom. The food industry likes to tell us that "one little cookie won't hurt you." While this is most likely true, the problem with eating that "one little cookie" is not how many points or calories it contains—but rather the fact that this infusion of sugar into the bloodstream, that ensues after eating it, is likely to set off the desire for more of the same later. Rather than focusing on the taste of this "delicious" cookie—by shifting your awareness to the likely result of now having to battle future cravings—it's much easier to say no to the cookie. The more you make this empowering choice, the less of a temptation these simple, processed carbs become. The trick is not to focus on being on any kind of diet, but rather on how good it feels to keep the mind-body clean and free. Also, it helps to know that if you really want a cookie, you can bake your own delicious and healthy treat using healthful ingredients such as whole oats and sesame seeds, and sweeteners such as coconut, golden raisins or prunes.

Creating a New Belief System

The only thing that could stop you from succeeding in making these internal shifts in your perceptions would be your belief that it's impossible for you to change. How do you change your beliefs? The first step is to become conscious of them. Ask yourself, do you think that it is possible for you to adopt new behaviors that reflect your intention to live a healthier life? If the answer is no, ask yourself why this is so. Write down your answers. Most likely, you will begin to list your liabilities as evidence that you could never fulfill your longing to be healthier and to be completely free from compulsion around food. Return to the preceding exercise, and ask yourself for proof that these arguments are incorrect. If you feel certain that you don't have the willpower necessary to radically change your perceptions and behaviors around food, write down the situations in your life that will convince you that you do, in fact, have willpower.

Recall incidents where you made up your mind to do something, and you knew that it was your destiny to accomplish it—and you did. Remember that it takes time to succeed in any endeavor, including changing your whole way of relating to yourself and food (or any addictive substance). Give yourself the gift of that time, while staying steadfast to the goal and gently self-correcting whenever you go astray. Soon your new way of thinking about yourself and food will become second nature.

The real issue is your need to know that you are worthy of what you desire. Perhaps you have everything you want in life besides this one thing—health and freedom in your relationship with food. Or there may be several areas in your life that you wish to improve. Can you look in the mirror and say to yourself, "I love you. You deserve to be happy"? Do that right now.

In the following exercise, you'll use affirmations as a powerful tool to access your deeper feelings. You'll also strengthen your connection to your heart's longing for fulfillment. As you become more aware of the underlying emotions that are driving your behavior, it will become easier to make new, healthier choices. Emotions are energy in motion and are always accompanied by not only the thought, but also the physical feeling, usually in the torso. So check your belly, solar plexus, chest, and even throat to see if there is a tightening or constriction there.

. . . .

EXERCISE: LEARNING TO LOVE YOURSELF

Go over to a mirror, look into your eyes, and tell yourself, "I love you, you deserve to be happy." Say, "I deserve to live at my ideal weight." Now breathe in and feel the response in your body. Pay attention to the feelings in your torso—your chest area, your solar plexus, and your lower belly. Continue to repeat this phrase to yourself slowly, each time breathing the sentences into the different parts of your body—your belly, your chest area (also known as your heart center), your pelvis, your throat, and your solar plexus. Notice how your body responds to your words, and allow yourself to have your experience without shutting it down. In other words, if you say those words into your throat, and you feel a lump rise up, allow the sadness to just be there without trying to censor or control it.

Awareness itself is healing, so send love and recognition to this part of your body. Just continue to speak the words softly and firmly into your being, including the places that are in pain. Often all those places need is some attention and acknowledgement. If there is a picture there in your throat that you become aware of, for example of a time when you couldn't speak your truth or were shut down, offer yourself compassion for that experience. Say to the younger you who had that experience, "I'm sorry that happened to you. I care about you. I love you. I respect you. You deserve to be happy."

Or perhaps, as you repeat the affirmations to yourself, you'll sense an expansion and a feeling of lightness in your chest. Open to receive this feeling, and notice what your body is saying to you. Perhaps the lightness and openness that you are feeling in your heart center is a sense of relief at being recognized and loved. Drink in that sensation, and feel your hunger to be appreciated.

Maybe there is a little girl or boy in your belly that's saying, "Really? Do you really mean that? Do you love me, and do I deserve to be happy?" It doesn't matter if you are the CEO of the largest bank in the world or the most distinguished politician in your country, within your belly is the less evolved part of yourself—the part of you that may have doubt or fear about what's possible. This part literally hungers for approval—and the approval has to come from you. It doesn't really matter what the outer world says about you, if you don't believe it and know it to be true in your heart. That goes for both positives and negatives.

If someone called you a banana peel, would it have any impact on you at all? Probably not, because there is no part of you that believes such a preposterous claim. But how much time do you waste believing negative ideas about yourself? Take a stand for the fact that you are the essence of love in your core. If you are unhappy with your consistent behaviors and the results they create in your life, realize that they are reoccurring because of your deep-seated belief that you are not worthy of something better.

The mirror exercise and affirming that you do love yourself—all parts of yourself—will help you to break such old, unproductive beliefs.

Do not underestimate the power within your affirmations. The spoken word has the ability to heal or to wound. The things that you tell yourself consistently shape your beliefs about what's true and what's possible. These beliefs then influence the behavioral choices you make daily, which create the big picture of your current reality.

When you do the mirror exercise, have some paper and different color pens nearby. Write down your positive affirmations in one color ink, and then write down your response to those affirmations in a different color. This way, when you go back and refer to these written statements, you'll easily be able to isolate the positive, constructive self-talk. Equally important, you'll see how, over time, your automatic responses to your internal dialogue shift. Continue to state and write the affirmations down, while noticing the physical reactions in your body, along with any statements that question the truth in your affirmations. Through continuous repetition of the positive statements, you will begin to wash away the deep-seated objections or blocks to accepting and receiving the greater good that awaits you. The act of writing the positive statements down helps to implant them even more deeply in the subconscious mind.

How to Identify Emotional Eating

What are the needs that you have been trying to meet by overeating or consistently selecting the wrong foods? Usually our needs fall into three categories. Beyond our need for physical sustenance—food, water, and shelter—we need love and compassion, safety and protection, and strength or power. These needs are biological and natural, however, when unexamined and operating unconsciously, these needs may cause us to act out in a way that is counterproductive. Let's take a look at each one.

The Need for Love

Our need for love and compassion stems from our desire to be connected with others, to feel good about ourselves, and to receive and give appreciation. We all want to feel valued, understood, and respected—to be heard, seen, and believed. Because of past hurts in your life, which may be triggered by things that are happening now, you may sometimes assume that you are not loved, respected, understood, or cared for. This could lead you to feel misunderstood, ashamed, guilty, embarrassed, heavy, unloved, rejected, sad, abandoned, lonely, or desperate. By feeling your feelings in the moment, you can discover what need is not being met.

For example, let's say that your husband commented that you are putting on some weight. You may react by feeling anger and respond, either aloud or to yourself, that he's not looking so good himself. You may want to inflict pain on him by ignoring him, or you may want to punish yourself because you know that his words are true. Perhaps you even find yourself heading toward the kitchen cabinet in search of leftover Halloween or Easter candy to help comfort you and soothe the pain you feel as a result of his words, as well as the reality that you have indeed put on weight. Or you may want to rebel against him. In that moment, ask yourself, "What need do I have that is underneath or behind this anger?" Sit with the anger for a few moments and notice where the sensation is in your body. No matter how strong it is, remind yourself that the sensation will pass and that it's not who you are.

If you are afraid that you will forget the present cause of your feelings and not take appropriate action because you are working with your feelings in this way, write down the scenario so that you can respond later when the tornado of your emotion has passed over.

For a moment, drop the story—meaning let go of the content of your thoughts to the best of your ability —and allow the feeling to be there without judging it or trying to change it and notice what else is there. Perhaps, behind the anger, you become aware of sadness. Allow yourself to feel the feeling. Ask yourself, "What am I needing?" You may be craving comfort, companionship, empathy, or nurturing. Resist the temptation to try to meet these needs through food. Give yourself what you truly need, instead. Ask yourself, "How can I get my need for support and kindness met?" Sit with it for a moment, and let your intuition show you your best course of action.

Maybe right now the best course of action is no action except sitting where you are and being with yourself and the sensations in your body. You may have the very pleasant surprise of discovering that as soon as you acknowledge to yourself what you really require—in this case love—your husband's remarks have minimal effect. Shower yourself with compassion as you recognize your need for love. Remind yourself that you already are loved, loving and loveable. You may even develop a feeling of compassion for him and his momentary insensitivity. Or perhaps you'll see how much he does love you and that he was simply expressing his concern for your health, happiness, and well-being. Perhaps he is actually self-conscious about his own weight! When you identify and fill your need for appreciation that was triggered by your feeling of anger, you will be able to deal with and respond to the current situation from a place of strength and insight.

The Need to Feel Safe

Another basic need that we all have is the need for safety and protection. Being fed and having enough to eat is a valid, innate need that we are all born with. Some of us may not have been fed enough as infants, and therefore, subconsciously, developed a feeling of being unsafe and are concerned whether we are going to have enough to eat, even though, rationally, we know that food is abundant and plentiful. If this subconscious feeling that there isn't or that there may in the future not be enough to eat is allowed to drive our behavior, it can wreak havoc on our life.

You may want a feeling of security, but is it what you really need? Perhaps having cabinets stocked with various types of cookies, chips, and soda pop gives you a feeling of security. When you tap into your true need for safety and protection, it becomes easier to discern that no amount of junk food could truly offer you that greater sense of being taken care of. Going to extreme measures to insure your own safety simply implies that you don't already have it. In reality, no amount of planning could assure your own safety. Ultimately, beyond the commonsense precautions we instinctively must take, each of us needs to cultivate a sense of trust regarding our physical safety and protection. When we realize that it's out of our hands and that the more we want a guarantee of safety, the more often it eludes us, we can begin to let go of the demand that we feel secure and trust that we are as safe and protected now as we were in our mother's womb.

While you are in the throes of the feeling, it's best that you take a moment to care for yourself. So feel the feeling that is coursing through your body and notice the physicality of the feeling inside you. Go inside and notice what is behind the sensation. Perhaps you are feeling afraid. As you move

into the sensation in your torso with your conscious awareness, you may become cognizant of a specific fear that you
won't have enough to eat. Ask yourself, "What am I needing
in this moment?" Breathe into the sensations that you are
feeling, and put space around them. Imagine a field of space
inside yourself and surrounding you. Write down or make a
mental note of what you truly desire.

Perhaps you require safety, comfort, food, shelter, security, nourishment, peace, air, water, sleep, or touch. Affirm to
yourself that you have everything you need. Say to yourself,
"All my needs are being met. I have everything I need." Look
at yourself in the mirror, and tell yourself those statements
in a peaceful, loving voice. If it is sleep that you are lacking,
lie down, even if you only have ten minutes. The benefit of a
short catnap can be incredible! If it's nourishment that you
need, imagine the various healthy foods that you could select
right now and see which one "lights up" for you. Perhaps a
delicious, crunchy carrot would satisfy you. Or maybe your
body is yearning for a piece of iron-rich meat to nourish your
blood. Go inside and pay attention to the signals that your
body is sending you.

If you see pictures of rich, chocolate brownies coming to
your mind, superimpose on them the fat on your body, or
the painful experience of eating such food regularly. If you
are tired a lot, imagine that those chocolate brownies are
what has gotten into your bloodstream and cells and made
you feel so exhausted, sapping the life force out of you. Use
your imagination to turn yourself off to the substances that
are poisoning you and sickening you. Go back inside and see
what your body really needs. If you really do want a carbohydrate, make it a complex carb—such as a baked potato or
some whole-grain pasta, but make sure to eat it in combination with healthy fat and protein.

The Need to Feel Powerful

Finally, we all have the need, or at least the desire, for some personal power over our life. How often do you find yourself seeking and demanding control? When we feel that our need to have control or power is being threatened, we may react by being pushy, demanding, or aggressive. Or we may respond by giving up, giving in, and feeling powerless. Either way, we are not acknowledging and filling our need for personal power in the world. The remedy for needing control is acceptance, surrender, and letting go.

It is common to find yourself in a power struggle with your children, spouse, or parents. This insatiable quest for control is nothing more than a veiled attempt to access your own personal power. Each of us needs to know that there is a force of strength and power within us, otherwise we would feel weak and incapable of surviving in this world. Instead of seeking control, we can begin to get in touch with the great foundation of strength and power that already resides within, at the core of our being. When you feel this pillar of force inside and begin to identify with it, you no longer need to assert and validate your power in ineffective, energy-draining ways.

Harnessing Your Own Resources

Through honoring and listening to your feelings, you can attain greater awareness and learn about yourself. When you feel the familiar bodily reactions—the tightening, bracing, and holding that goes along with any power struggle—give yourself space to breathe through what you are experiencing. Ask yourself, "What am I needing?" Aside from space, you may be longing for solitude, courage, freedom, clarity, expression, ease, autonomy, or choice. Honor what you are discovering about your needs. Take time to be with yourself so that you can find ways to fill your needs without returning to harmful eating habits. Sometimes just looking in the mirror and acknowledging what you need is all it takes to free you from feeling out of control. Affirm to yourself, "I am in control. I let go of this power struggle." Look in the mirror and tell yourself, "I love you. I respect you. I am lovable, loving and loved," "I am confident in myself," "I have the right to feel confident and self-assured." Letting go does not mean that you are giving up. It simply means that you are turning the matter over to your higher wisdom and creativity, which you are entrusting to come up with a solution.

Wanting and demanding outside approval, security, and control implies that you are in some way deficient. Getting in touch with the deeper resources inside yourself—the strength, love, courage, and innate protection—will help you to associate with the deeper parts of yourself and give to your outer self what you are truly craving. When you state your affirmations, practice declaring them in the first person: "I am loved," "I am safe," "I am powerful and in control," "I feel confident," "I am grateful." Feel how proclaiming the affirmations in this way makes them real for you and helps you to get in touch with the strength and goodness that exist within your true essence.

The more you give to yourself from your deeper self, the easier it becomes to look behind the outer circumstances of your life situation and identify with the immense potential for love and possibility inside yourself. In the next chapter, you will begin to discover and explore your personal power and deeper resources even more. You can increasingly begin to identify with the deeper parts of yourself that are available to help you fill all your needs, and release the habit of using food, substances or alcohol in unhealthy ways that drain your precious life force.

4. What Voice Are You Listening To?

Realize that everything you are seeking is already inside of you. It is simply not accessible at the level in which you have been looking. Each of us has many levels to our being. On the outer level is the personality, the ego, the conscious, analytical mind. This is often the part of yourself that you are most identified with, even though it is the most limiting. In fact, we tend to see life through the lens of the outer layer of the self.

The Conscious Mind

The conscious mind generally has many opinions about ourself and others that it takes for granted to be true. It may believe, for example, that we are destined to be fat or to have no control over our life and our eating habits. The outer layer of the self has many likes and dislikes, and most of all wants gratification—usually instantly. The ego, personality, or outer layer of the self will say things like "I deserve to eat that," "I want that," and "I definitely don't want to be deprived." The personality may contain pictures, ideas, or images about what it means to eat healthy food. Consistently eating nutritious foods in moderate amounts may seem boring or tedious to the outer layer of the self. This is why if we are dieting as a result of an impulse from the outer layer of the self, it's impossible to succeed because the whole mentality is one of struggle for a short-term gain. The self thinks that it is the body and mind only, and it wants what it wants. The voice of the self often sounds like this:

"I can't stop eating chocolate." "I have no willpower."

"You only live once. I want to enjoy my life." "I don't have the discipline it takes to eat differently."

"Healthy food is boring."

"I'm not going to eat what 'they' want me to eat."

"I'll always be tired. Therefore I need caffeine and simple carbohydrates for energy."

"I'll just die if I have to give up snack food." "This is going to be very hard."

"It's too complicated to try to take care of myself."

"I won't be able to change."

"I'm sure that I'll fail. I've always failed before." "What's the point of working so hard to change my eating habits, when I know I'll just end up going back to my old ways eventually?"

"The pain that I will endure to create change will only bring temporary reward."

"I'm dreading the effort I have to make."

The voice of the self can be extremely convincing, and you may often feel tempted to stop with that voice and follow it, without exploring a deeper truth. The voice of the self is often echoed by the doubts and fears of your friends and family and confirmed by your life's events or the experiences of those around you.

Your conscious mind desires health, but it also wants to fit in with the crowd and take the easier road. Sometimes, though, what appears to be the easier road is actually the path that takes you away from what your deepest heart desires, and ultimately causes suffering. One aspect of the voice of the self is the voice of fear, which uses phrases such as, "you'll always be weak," or "you'll never change," or it makes unfair comparisons between you and fictitious people such as, "so-and-so would never react the way you do." The voice of fear creates an internal environment of feeling "less than" or not good enough or somehow defective. Unfortunately, the voice is often compelling and clever, and it plays on our greatest weakness or insecurities about ourselves. If we follow that dialogue, it can take us very far from our own core of essential goodness.

Sometimes we get so used to the voice of fear that we don't even question it. So when it tells us, "That is so awful that you just ate those cookies. You are completely hopeless. You might as well just eat the whole box," we often don't inquire about the validity of what the voice is asserting and give it authority that it doesn't deserve.

Often the fearful place inside of you doesn't know that it will always have access to food. The negative voice urges you to eat it all now, because there won't be any later. Or if you have a history of dieting, part of you fears that the next time you decide to go on a diet, you will starve yourself and be unable to eat the foods that you love.

It is human nature to want to eat more if you don't know when you'll have the opportunity to eat again. If you are used to ignoring your body's hunger signals, then your body stops trusting that you will feed it again when it's hungry. Your inner voices will play on this fear by encouraging you to "grab it while you can." If you came from a big family where there wasn't always enough food to go around, this self-sabotaging mentality may be deeply engrained in your psyche.

The Inner Self

The self-talk that leads us to freedom from the limited thinking of the past is the voice of our own essence behind the incessant chatter of the conscious mind—the voice of love, compassion, and wisdom. This is the voice of your own inner truth—the voice that does know and want what's best for you. It comes from the core of your being, from which your greatest qualities emanate. The more you begin to trust this deeper, wiser voice, the more acting in accordance with it will become a positive habit. This affirmative voice can let you know about your higher potential and the greater reality that's possible for you. This wise part of yourself knows that the negative eating habits you engage in can be broken in an instant. Getting in touch with your inner self at your core is essential for realizing your intention and continuing to build your self-esteem.

This intelligent voice beckons to you always, but it's often quieter than the constant monologue of the voices of self and fear, so you need to listen closely. If you do pay attention, you will hear it whispering to you words of love and comfort and deep wisdom. The wisest part of you knows that you are using food as a way to avoid feelings, to fill inner needs, and to distract or comfort yourself, and it is always there to soothe you and give you love. It also patiently waits for you to open to this love. It's very polite and does not force itself on you. Listening to and following the voice of love and truth takes practice and, with time, becomes a new way of living. As long as you are alive, you will continue to hear from the voices of self and fear, but more and more you can increase your faith that the voice of love and truth is also present behind those voices, and is here to feed you and give you the real medicine—that which your heart and soul is searching for.

True happiness and lasting freedom from food addiction can only be found when you open to the loving voice inside the core of your being. Otherwise, the voices of self and fear are sure to sabotage your efforts along the way. The voice of truth is the wise part of you that will help you to let go of any mistakes of the past. When you stop covering over this precious aspect of yourself with food and more food, it becomes easier to make contact with this place. You can make it your mission to live from this deeper, more solid place inside yourself. You may recall the inner whispering reassuring you, at some time in your life, "Everything is OK, you are perfect just as you are, even with your imperfections," or "Don't eat that, darling, it will make you sick." Using the skills you learned in Chapter 3, you can strengthen this deeper aspect of yourself by affirming, "You are loved," "You deserve to feel happy and confident." You can make a conscious decision to start taking this voice seriously and follow its beckoning.

Open yourself to the truth of your greater nature that will take you far beyond the desires and pain experienced by the outer self. Even if you don't feel it right now, trust that a wiser, vaster part of you is within. Even if you doubt it, act as if it exists. The more you can identify with your deeper nature—the love that you are—the more you will be able to embody it and let your outer body reflect the love and beauty in your deep heart. When you finally get in touch with the personal power you carry, you will know at a very deep level, with a sense of certainty, the preciousness that you carry.

Once this knowledge becomes your driving force, breaking free from the grip of uncontrollable sugar cravings will be easy and natural, and your addictions will fall away effortlessly. This is why, for long-term success, it is imperative for you to discover the deeper layers of your being by seeking to uncover and fill your true desires.

To understand the connection between the various parts or levels of our self, it's helpful to imagine that each of us is a vast ocean. We can relate to ourselves from the point of view of the waves on the surface or the huge depths. The waves are the continuous chatter and judgments of the conscious mind. The depths of the ocean of your heart are undisturbed by this chatter of the intellect or by all the memories, automatic behaviors, and functions of the subconscious, which are just under the waves. At the bottom of this ocean is a quiet, still place within you where there is only peace, only love. As you travel further into your inner heart, you will feel your connection to the part of you that's far greater than the unproductive programming that may currently be running your life. The depths of your being are endless. As you practice the Break-Your-Craving-State Technique that you'll learn in Chapter 7, you can start to travel to the places within yourself that generate freedom and happiness—and lead a more meaningful life. You don't have to continue to be tossed around by every wave on the ocean of life. Instead, you can cruise through the deeper levels like a submarine.

Getting in Touch with Your Inner Self

How do you travel to the deeper layers of your being and get a taste of this deeper part of yourself? Perhaps you have been fortunate enough to have experienced a spontaneous witnessing of a higher part of yourself and felt a sense of oneness and connection with all of life. Often after the death of a loved one a person may ask for a sign from his or her beloved and receive one so clear that it's impossible to deny its reality. In that moment it becomes undeniable that life is a much greater mystery than our conscious mind can fathom. Maybe you experienced a higher bliss or peace when participating in a sport or creating music or art. Perhaps there has been a time when you lost all sense of time and life took on a surreal, still, and beautiful quality—despite any suffering that may have been present. It's like getting a glimpse into the higher realms of life, beyond the world of thought.

I experienced such spontaneous bliss most vividly when my daughters were born. Prior to that I never had consciously known such a profound love. I remember just looking at my newborn baby, my eyes welling up with tears, in awe of the miracle that had just occurred and filling up with the deepest gratitude I had known, knowing that this gift—this love—was for me. When we are fortunate enough to have moments when we experience complete bliss and unity with life—perhaps hiking in a majestic spot in nature—we have the opportunity to open our perception and step into a greater reality.

Unfortunately, many of us get scared and begin to doubt that the experience even occurred, or rationalize it as an unusual psychic event and just go back to living in the "real world" and eating "real food." What if the real world—filled with the angst of having to perform or look a certain way, not being good enough, and needing to measure up to some ridiculous image of outer beauty—was the world that is actually an illusion? What if the inner world of deep love, truth, and strength was the world that we were really meant to rely on? What if all we had to do was open to that reality more and more in order to experience all that our heart desires? What if living at your ideal weight and being free of diet pill, caffeine, alcohol and/or sugar addiction had nothing to do with willpower and dieting, but only with aligning with the force of greater intelligence and love that always intended for you to eat natural foods and lead an active and rested, balanced lifestyle? Once we make this connection, the means—the way to achieve balance in our moods and energy level naturally, in a healthy way—is revealed to us and becomes second nature, and at the same time the unhealthy addictions and habits melt away.

Letting Change Come from the Inside

Do you have to force yourself to take a shower? No, it's natural to shower or bathe regularly because you enjoy the feeling of cleanliness and presenting yourself to the world feeling fresh and clean. Once you start connecting with the deeper levels of your being, you will naturally wish to eat the foods that come from the earth, that will bring you health and vitality, and at the same time fill yourself up with pure, clean water and life-giving oxygen. You'll get back in touch with the natural joy of movement that you came into this world with and free yourself from the prison of a sedentary lifestyle.

When your motivation to lose weight and eliminate unproductive habits and addiction is sparked by your deep desire to honor your life as well as your commitment to live in the highest way possible for you, in the precious time that you have here on earth, you will naturally take on the behaviors that will lead to a healthy, fit body. When you realize the greater potential for your life, you'll no longer have to force yourself to exercise or give up chocolate. You'll intrinsically gravitate toward the water-rich foods that support your life. You'll naturally want to move and celebrate your very existence—perhaps through dance, walking, or even simply stretching. When you continue to set your intention daily, as you learned to do in Chapter 1, from the deepest part of yourself that you can access, you are given everything you need—the tools, wisdom, and inner power—to bring this heartfelt desire to fruition.

Accessing Love for Yourself

The person who stands in front of the mirror fretting about her weight and feeling guilty about the food she wants to eat or has eaten may seem to say to you that this is the sum total of who you are. No matter how convincing she is, you will soon discover that—though she is real—this limited you is only a fragment of who you essentially are. This you who suffers the consequences of food addiction is your physical, outer self. She is your small self—your ego—who thinks, feels, and acts and appears to be running the show. Although at this time they may not be in your awareness, beyond this outer level of your being are the deeper parts of yourself where the opportunity to create real, lasting change lies.

If you are unsure about whether there really is a deeper part of yourself that is made of love and beauty, see yourself as a child. Or, if there is a child in your life whom you adore, let that special child be a mirror of who you truly are. Like a dirty mirror, your true self—your loving heart—has been covered over with doubt, fear, and unproductive programming that causes you to sabotage yourself. Don't keep adding layers of dirt to the mirror. Instead, no matter where you currently are in your life, begin to clean it off.

When you look at yourself as an innocent baby, ask yourself whether you would treat that beautiful child the way you treat yourself. If you have negative, judging thoughts about your adult self, imagine how difficult it would be to project those same condemning judgments on this small, innocent baby who is essentially a part of you. As you make contact with the infant that you were when you entered this world—and realize that this innocent soul is who you really are—it becomes more difficult to be so hard on yourself and take actions that are harmful to you.

Where Do My Cravings Come From?

The thoughts that you choose to listen to, in addition to your mental images, program your subconscious mind. The subconscious is like a computer that's programmed by your repetitive thinking, strong emotions, and inner pictures. If our minds were an iceberg, the conscious part would be the tip, and the subconscious would be the vast majority of the iceberg. Locked within the subconscious part of our minds are the habits we have had, often since childhood, and all the automatic behaviors that basically run our lives. If every time we are feeling stressed, we reach for the cookies, this pattern becomes deeply ingrained in the subconscious part of the mind.

The thoughts and habits keep us functioning on autopilot. The more we continue with the same destructive behaviors, the more natural they feel—almost as if reaching for the cookies were an intrinsic part of who we are, despite the negative results over the long term. If we are convinced that we need a muffin and a cup of coffee to get us going in the morning, this certainly becomes true for us. The subconscious mind controls most of the activities and thoughts that we engage in throughout the day, and often we find ourselves repeating the same thoughts and behaviors over and over without conscious consideration.

The subconscious part of our mind gets its signals from the outer environment, such as the clock on the wall, and our conscious interpretations—deciding it's time to eat. So, for example, if the conscious mind decides that it wants to devour a big, greasy hero sandwich, the subconscious will create the desire. As the image, taste, smell, and feeling of eating the oversized sandwich gains momentum in the subconscious, you're likely to have the urge to act on this notion immediately.

The subconscious mind does not care if the programming that's running makes any sense at all—it is simply operating automatically, based on the current program that has been installed. Until you change the program, you are at the mercy of the old habitual reactions from the past, many of which are undoubtedly keeping you trapped in addictive and compulsive behavior that is chipping away at the quality of your life. By choosing the voice of the wise heart instead of the voices of doubt and fear, you can begin to install a new set of beliefs into your subconscious mind. These new beliefs can lead you to a much healthier and happier relationship with food and with yourself.

Listening to Your Deeper Self

One way to begin to discern between the various voices and their impact on you is to notice what part of your body they are coming from. You may assume that your internal self-talk is all generated in your head, and many times it is. However, if you tune in to your body, your awareness will be enhanced. For example, I may have a voice in my head encouraging me to eat that last doughnut in the box. I may then become aware of another voice that has a shaming quality to it that retorts, "No, don't do that. You'll get even fatter. You've already gained so much weight."

As you cringe at the nasty tone of the guilt-inducing admonition, stop and open your awareness. Because fear and doubt often come from the belly, you may realize that there is a tightening in your gut that is not only a reaction to the hurtful comment, but also the place from which that statement originated. Alternatively, you may notice that the voice of fear is coming from outside yourself and speaking to you in the second person. Recognize that the voice is not who you are and that it is simply there as a way to test your inner resolve to live to a higher potential. Make the decision to stop feeding the fear by not giving energy to concerns such as "Am I good enough?" or "Am I strong enough?"

Instead, listen for the third, quieter, subtler voice, which is likely to be emanating from your heart. It may be speaking very softly, tenderly letting you know that "Doughnuts are always going to be around, whether this is the last one in the box today or not. You deserve a better life that doesn't revolve around toxic, processed foods. Drink some water, and have some fruit with cheese, if you are hungry. You are worthy. Care for yourself."

Hear the gentleness and truthfulness in this wiser, more

caring voice. Feed your own heart (not your belly) by giving it love. When your heart is full, it naturally feeds your tummy and all parts of you with the love they are crying out for. See your inner beauty. The more you recognize your inner beauty, the better you will treat yourself.

Tuning In to Your Deeper Wisdom

It's amazing how out of touch we can be with our own body— barely aware that our shoes are squeezing our feet, or that our pants are so tight we can hardly breathe. It's time to start really noticing and feeling what is happening to ourselves physically. Your deep, wise, intuitive voice guides you toward a life of health and happiness. This quiet place within encourages you to feed yourself—to give yourself permission to eat, but choose your foods wisely. When you tune in to it, the wisdom inside you shows you how to get in touch with your body by feeling and noticing when your stomach is full. Your wise self encourages you to pause when you are eating and notice how full you are feeling. Pay attention and sense the signals of fullness. Honor your body, and when your stomach is full, stop eating.

Before I learned to listen to my body, I used to eat all the time, not because I was hungry, but just because I wanted to. My body became completely out of balance because I was eating whatever I wanted, whenever I wanted, having no respect for the kinds of foods my body actually needed and thrived on. When you live this way, as I did, it may seem like all of a sudden, your whole system is completely out of whack, and you may be tempted to take some desperate measure that will suppress your symptoms—such as drinking alcohol or reaching for a drug to restore yourself to health and well-being. This may bring temporary relief, but is likely to do little to rectify the cause of your problem. When I began to learn to eat more moderately, in a healthy way, I could feel a natural rhythm to what my body required. By learning to discern and listen to my body's hunger signals, I actually became less hungry and less susceptible to food cravings.

As you fill your deeper needs by following your inner voice of truth, you will no longer find yourself filled with insatiable cravings and appetites. It is absolutely possible to enjoy food and be completely satisfied with the healthy foods that you are eating. After experimenting with your options, you also may decide to limit your food choices purposely, without feeling like you are on a diet, simply because it helps to break cravings. This will only work, in the long run, if you come to this conclusion by examining the evidence presented by your voice of truth—not the voice of self or fear.

That aspect of the voice of the outer self that is the voice of fear may appear to have the same goal as the voice of love: to get you to improve your eating habits and stop overeating the wrong foods. However, there is a huge difference in their motivation. The voice of fear and doubt wants you to be ashamed of yourself and your behavior, feel awful, and guiltily make a new choice. That only works over the short run.

The voice of love, however, is sympathetic to you and compassionate and sees what you are going through. It seeks to gently remind you how eating certain foods makes you feel—to notice the effect the foods you are eating have on your body. The loving part of you desires so much more for you and knows without a doubt that there is a world of good waiting for you. It sees your difficulty, your challenges and struggles, and hears the inner voices that are hurtful to you. With all this understanding, it seeks to inform you about a greater reality—a deeper truth—that can free you from the type of life you have been living. It knows that you are simply repeating old patterns and habits that no longer serve you. It wants to wake you up from the dream and help you to see that you can have everything that you want and more, if only you believe it to be true and ask for it by setting a deep intention to have it and following through with yourself.

The reason you need to access the voice of your heart, as opposed to allowing yourself to be ruled by the never-ending chatter of the mind, is because it is only by changing your thoughts that you can ultimately change your behavior. Simply trying to alter your actions doesn't work. How many times have you tried to "just stop" reaching for candy bars during a stressful day? Or tried to get yourself to not eat bread or chips at night? The reason these strategies don't work is that it is almost impossible to change your behavior if you don't first change the thoughts that precede it.

However, you have probably also discovered that changing thoughts isn't necessarily easy. You may have told yourself that you are just not going to think about ice cream. Of course, ice cream, then, probably moved to the center of your consciousness. The only way to really alter thoughts, over the long run, is to change the perceptions that precede the thoughts. You can do that by learning to look through the lens of the heart, not the lens of the ego, the limited mind.

Two Key Words to Reprogram Your Mind

Rather than increasing the enticement of a certain food by telling yourself that you're not allowed to eat it (the voice of the self and doubt), use the power within your mind to convince yourself that you don't *want* to eat it. How do you do that? The key word is *because*. I don't want to eat this food now or ever *because* it makes me feel____. You fill in the blank. For me, I don't want to eat cake or candy ever *because* it makes me feel tired, irritable, and like I'll never have enough. It upsets the quality of my life *because* it turns all my thoughts and desires to food. It tricks me into thinking that's all that there is and that this is a source of happiness. From experience, I know this is not true. It is actually a source of deep pain that I no longer wish to subject myself to.

Now ask yourself, "What do I want *instead*?" For me, *instead*, I want and choose freedom from compulsion around food. I choose regular, moderate exercise, which makes me feel fabulous. I love to get up early and walk on the beach. I love to spend time writing and helping others to lose weight and make positive changes in their lives. I love the deep relaxation of my body and mind that comes from meditation. I prefer to take time every day to deeply rest, instead of reaching for food every time I feel tired.

Giving up food addiction or bad eating habits frees me to truly enjoy the time I spend with my husband, myself, children, and friends without obsessing about the foods I am or am not eating. It frees me up to focus on and create my life's purpose. The *because* is essential to your long-term success, as is the *instead* statement that follows it.

Writing these statements down on paper will solidify them much more than simply making a mental note of them, and I encourage you to take the time to do so. Remember that when your intention is hooked into your motivation (which comes from the *because* and the *instead*) from the deepest part of your being—your inner wisdom—your subconscious mind will accept your command readily and make it so. Your inner wisdom doesn't shame you into making healthier choices, but it helps you to change your perspective so that you actually prefer a new, healthier style of eating and caring for yourself.

. . . .

EXERCISE: INCREASING YOUR MOTIVATION

Take a moment and write down your reasons for wanting to eliminate the foods that are harmful to you. Use the following format:

I don't want to eat this food now or ever

because it makes me feel ____.

Instead I choose ____.

Make a list of all the reasons why you are determined to update your eating behaviors and the new choices you are making instead.

Write Down What You Hear

Because your subconscious mind runs on programming, the voices that you listen to consistently become habitual and can be difficult to detect. The voice of truth and love is the voice we have the most difficulty tuning in to because we are not used to it. Because it is softer and subtler, it is often drowned out by the loud, dominating voice of fear. So the next time you are bombarded with voices of insecurity, weakness, or negativity, listen for the softer voice within that dispels the darkness by turning on the light.

Don't stop with the outer voices—keep looking and

listening for what is deeper and truer. Let the voice of the inner judge and jury that seeks to inform you whether you are being "good" or "bad" know that it is no longer in control of you. When you hear that fearful voice authoritatively asserting that your choices are "permissible" or "forbidden," know the truth inside yourself—that the real issue is simply how the foods you eat and the drinks or substances you consume impact your body. Stand up to that voice by writing down its words. Writing the words down will help give you some distance because it separates you from their effect.

. . . .

EXERCISE: NOT STOPPING WITH OUTER VOICES

Think about a time when you engaged in unproductive eating behavior. What voice was present when you first began to eat? Recall your inner dialogue and write it down. Notice where in your body each voice comes from, and map out where it will lead you if you listen to it.

Spend a moment focusing on your heart center and listen for a deeper, kinder, more subtle voice. Write it down, and ask yourself where it will lead you if you listen.

Your wise internal voice is your inner teacher that wants you to believe that what you want is possible. Your belief that it's not achievable is a result of limited information, based on your past. As you allow yourself to be reinformed by your wise self that has new, updated information, you will see that your beliefs begin to shift. When you finally believe that within you is the power to shape your destiny, you will get in touch with the inner resources that can help you take control of this area of your life. This will lead you to experience the changes you most desire in your life—you'll see it when you believe it.

When you decide and commit to living in a new way, you will be able to master this area of your life where you have felt weak or out of control in the past. This is quite different from preferring that things would be different some day. Your new beliefs will fuel new, more desirable actions, since all action is preceded by thought. It's not wishful thinking, but rather harnessing your inner resources and committing to new actions daily. It's not what you do once in a while that will impact your life profoundly, but it's what you do consistently that will shape the ultimate destiny of your lifelong relationship with food.

On the outer level, your voice of self may have you convinced that you are helpless and weak-willed in this area of your life. By committing to yourself and to searching inside for deeper truths with new supporting evidence, you will find yourself moving in the direction of freedom from lifelong patterns of self-destructiveness around food.

5. Breathing for Energy and Health

Your body and mind need oxygen to thrive. Although we aren't usually consciously aware of how we are breathing, staying connected to the voice of the outer self often keeps us in a state of shallow chest breathing. By contrast, when we begin to drop out of our heads and move into our hearts, we may find that our breathing becomes fuller and deeper. In this chapter you'll learn how breathing properly will help you stay attuned to the voice of your inner self.

Shallow breathing all these years has deprived your cells of vital oxygen and nutrients, affecting both your physical and emotional health. Unconscious breath holding slowly chips away at the quality of your life, leading to fatigue, depression, anxiety, and a host of physical ailments. Shallow breathing, in addition to providing less oxygen to your body, actually severs the tie between you and your emotions because taking in a smaller amount of oxygen leads to feeling less. In this way, shallow breathing and eating processed junk food with wild abandon have a similar negative result. Though both superficial chest breathing and overeating foods that are toxic to your system successfully keep you from fully experiencing your painful feelings, they also keep you from experiencing true joy and aliveness, and ultimately lead to even stronger states of depression, fatigue, and anxiety. This keeps alive the vicious cycle of not wanting to breathe fully or stop eating the offending foods, because if you did, you might have to feel the unwanted emotions.

When you stop a feeling by holding your breath or by stuffing it with sugar, you are in essence cutting yourself off from your life force. This can lead to feelings of aloneness, separation, sadness, jitteriness, or nervousness. Naturally, if you're like most people, you'll want to get rid of these unpleasant feelings as soon as possible, and thus perpetuate the cycle of shallow breathing along with addiction to sugar, caffeine, and alcohol.

The Physical Benefits of Oxygen

As you take time to practice the breathing exercises in this chapter every day, for a minimum of ten to fifteen minutes, you will begin to put an end to this harmful chain of events. Your energy will begin to increase as you feed your body with the vital oxygen that it requires in order to thrive. As you get used to exhaling deeply and fully through your mouth, you will cleanse your system of toxins and carbon dioxide. When your energy increases through the deep breathing, you will find it easier to incorporate physical activity and deep rest into your daily life. The combination of breathing fully, resting deeply, and exercising your body physically will restore your body to a new level of health, vigor, and vitality. Once you experience this feeling of being truly alive, you will naturally wish to honor and care for your body by feeding it only the foods that are sustaining your life and nourishing you in mind, body, emotion, and spirit.

One of the most powerful tools for internal change is the breath. As simple as it is, the breath, the vital force that keeps us alive, also has the ability to completely shift our level of consciousness when we open to new ways to experience this natural part of our existence. We can spend our whole life breathing unconsciously—being breathed—or we can direct our conscious mind to the breath and learn a lot about ourselves in the process.

It can be quite enlightening to begin to notice your natural breathing rhythm throughout the day. It may come as a surprise to you to observe how often you may be holding your breath or barely breathing at all. Many of us live in a way that keeps our bodies keyed up and ready to react to the influx of incoming stressors that we are often barraged with. Subconsciously, you may resist relaxation, instead bracing yourself for the inevitable stressors of life that you anticipate on the horizon. If you are like most of my clients, you may often find yourself in a state of heightened arousal, addicted to the rush of chemicals being released into your body from the regular stress of life on your adrenal glands. The great news is that once you make the connection that even though your habits are medicating your "sick" condition, they are also, in reality, perpetuating the painful cycle of addiction that is preventing you from living fully, you have the freedom to make a new choice.

Chest Breathing Is Stress Breathing

One way to make your way of life and its effect on your body and your food choices more apparent is to begin to tune in to your breath, without trying to change it. When you realize that shallow chest breathing is stress breathing and that deep abdominal breathing creates the opposite response—generating a relaxation response within—you will begin to make the important mind-body connection that will give you new choices. If you watch a baby or a cat breathing, you will notice that it is breathing deep into its belly, allowing the breath to fill its whole body. This is the easy, full breath of relaxation—of fully being in the moment with life.

However, it doesn't take long for a small child to start reacting to the stressors in its environment, or adopt the breathing patterns of its caretakers, and make the switch to chest breathing. Shallow breathing or breath holding is a direct response to stress. It is actually a protective mechanism, because it prevents us from experiencing our emotions. Remember our emotions are energy in motion, and holding the breath stops that flow of energy. So it certainly works for stifling the painful emotions that we all encounter as we progress through life. When you hold your breath, you stop the feeling. The only downside is that doing so creates extreme stress in the body and only exacerbates the difficult feelings that we are trying so desperately to suppress. When we hold our breath or barely breathe, the negative feelings of sadness, frustration, anger, or jealousy do not disappear, but only become repressed and will have to be dealt with later in one way or another. In the same way, many times we reach for food as a way to submerge our feelings. Shallow breathing and overeating or bingeing on sweets and carbs go hand-in-hand with repression of emotion.

For example, imagine as a small child that your parent got angry with you and yelled at you. You cowered in fear and instinctively made your breathing shallow. You didn't want to feel the pain in your body that resulted from being the recipient of your parent's disappointment. By stopping the full flow of your breath, you were able to successfully stop the energy. However, because the fear in you was not fully experienced and resolved, it stayed in your body in the form of an energy block. Perhaps later in life, your wife or husband got upset with you because you're frequently home late for dinner. Your spouse's annoyance then triggered the same feelings in you that you felt as a child when your parent yelled at you.

Again you hold your breath unconsciously, and this time, vaguely aware of the discomfort in your body caused by the stuck energy and oxygen deprivation, you seek to gratify yourself with a beer or some blueberry pie to change the way you are feeling. This perpetuates the pattern of reacting to stress by stopping the energy of your emotions with shallow breathing and turning to food (or any other substance) to comfort yourself. Although holding the breath does serve the positive outcome of keeping the negative feelings at bay, unfortunately, it only creates a far less desirable result in the long run. Not only will suppressed feelings lead to over-eating, bingeing, and craving the wrong foods to help numb the lingering discomfort, but they can also cause disease or illness in the mind and body.

Awareness Is the Key

The solution to this type of very common pattern is to become aware of the way that you are breathing. Just the awareness alone will help your breathing shift to a healthier pattern. A healthier pattern means taking fuller, deeper, diaphragmatic breaths.

The diaphragm is the dome-shaped muscle that separates the belly from the chest. When we breathe deeply and correctly, the breath pushes the diaphragm muscle down, and the abdominal and intestinal organs are massaged by the breath, which creates optimum health for your digestive and eliminative systems. This kind of breathing is contrary to how so many of us were taught to hold the stomach in. With healthful belly breathing, we take the breath deep into our lungs, pushing the stomach out and filling our lungs all the way up with life-giving oxygen. The oxygen we take in with the breath and the carbon dioxide we expel with the exhalation energize the body and sustain life. The more efficiently we learn to breathe, the more energy and vitality we naturally have, and therefore the higher quality of life we experience.

Also, once you develop the habit of breathing more fully and completely, you will be able to do so in all situations, including stressful life events, ending your need to cope with everyday upsets by gorging on unhealthy food. The negative feelings that you have been running away from will be experienced more fully as sensations moving through your body, and you will more easily be able to return to a state of equilibrium, control, and peacefulness.

Rather than expecting yourself to breathe calmly, easily, and fully in the face of upsetting events, understand that the more frequently you practice the technique of deep, meditative breathing, the easier it will be to employ the method when you are under duress. Set up a system for yourself in which you can check your breathing periodically throughout the day. You can use the alarm on your watch or put a sticker near the phone or a sign in your bathroom or car that says, "breathe." Remember to take full, deep breaths throughout the day. In fact, I recommend that you take twenty to forty full, deep breaths as you go through the course of your daily routine. In addition, practice the following exercise for at least ten to fifteen minutes twice every day; find a quiet place where you will not be disturbed. Before you begin, get comfortable.

. . . .

EXERCISE: BREATHING MEDITATION FOR DEEP RELAXATION

1. Lie down on the floor or bed and close your eyes. Place your hand on your chest and begin to breathe normally. Feel the sensation of your breath—your life force—without making any effort on your part.

2. Notice your breath and how deep it feels. Be aware of any thoughts in your mind, and very gently bring your awareness back to your breath.

3. Imagine a screen in front of you. On the screen, see the word *stillness* written in golden-white light. Allow the word to float off the screen and enter into you, resting underneath your hand that is placed on your chest.

4. Breathe the word *stillness* deeper into your chest, and allow your whole body to relax and sink down into the floor or bed.

5. Move your hand down to your upper belly and feel your breath dropping down. Allow your breath to fill you even more fully. Take a few full, complete breaths with your hand near your solar plexus.

6. Now move your hand down to your lower belly near your pelvis, and imagine your breath filling your whole torso with stillness.

7. Finally, imagine that your breath is like a warm caress, touching you deeply and gently filling you with the life force and loving, healing energy.

This breathing exercise will help you transfer the benefits into your daily life. Then, when you get the urge for some chocolate, you'll be able to take some deep, breaths, center yourself, and feel what your body truly needs.

The Moment of Stillness

The quietest, most sublime period of the breath cycle is the moment after exhalation, just before the next inhalation. It can be very helpful to tune in to that moment, as this is a time when true relaxation occurs in the body. To help you discover this peaceful place for yourself, take a deep breath in through your nose to the count of ten and hold it. Now exhale out your mouth with a big sigh. Wait a moment before you take the next breath, and just feel that moment of stillness. If you are unsure about it, repeat the exercise. Just before your next inhalation is a wonderful time to relax your muscles completely. The more you are able to focus on your breathing and feel the sensation of calm that deep inhaling and exhaling generates, the easier it will become to relax your entire body. As the tension in your muscles begins to let go, you will no doubt experience a greater freedom, which can lead you to a wider variety of choices regarding your diet and lifestyle.

Much of your unhealthy food, alcohol or substance cravings is simply a distortion of your hunger for energy. You need energy to live, and one way or another your body has to get it in order to survive. Once you experience the incredible boost of energy that comes from power breathing coupled with physical exercise, you'll no longer need to turn to unhealthy eating and lifestyle patterns in a feeble attempt to energize yourself. As the awareness of your breath cycle increases throughout the day and you begin to experience the benefit of full, complete breathing, you can begin to incorporate some power breathing exercises into your day. Here are some simple breathing exercises to increase energy:

Breathing Exercises

EXERCISE: ALTERNATE NOSTRIL BREATHING

Sit comfortably with your spine straight. Close off your right nostril with your right thumb. While slowly counting to eight, inhale through your left nostril. Hold your breath to the count of four. Now close off your left nostril with your right index finger and exhale out of your right nostril to the count of eight. Now, keeping your left nostril closed off with your right index finger, breathe in through your right nostril to the count of eight. Hold it to the count of four. Exhale out of your left nostril to the count of eight as you close your right nostril with your right thumb. Continue for several minutes. Rest and breathe normally, maintaining a heightened awareness of your breath reaching your belly.

EXERCISE: THE COUNTING BREATH

Take a deep breath in and exhale fully and completely. Now inhale slowly while counting mentally from one to four. Hold the breath to the count of eight. Now exhale slowly to the count of sixteen. Repeat four times. If this is challenging for you, begin by inhaling to the count of four, holding for the count of four, and exhaling to the count of eight. Experiment with breathing in and out through your nose. Alternatively, you can inhale through your nose and exhale through your mouth.

Variation: Inhale while counting to four and hold the breath to the count of four. Now exhale to the count of four and pause to the count of four. Repeat the cycle.

. . . .

EXERCISE: BREATHING AND ENERGIZING

Lie down in a comfortable position on the floor or bed. As you inhale, imagine that you are breathing through all the pores of your skin. Inhale fully and imagine that you are breathing energy, life, light, and vitality fully into your body. Visualize with every slow, deep inhalation your cells being filled and recharged with energy and expansive light.

Now with each exhalation imagine that you are sending this vitality—this light— out into the universe. Breathing in and out through the whole surface of your skin, feel yourself receiving light and energy as you inhale and radiating it out to the world as you exhale. With every breath you take, your brightness and radiance is increasing, as you breathe through all the pores of your skin. You are receiving energy and love through your breath and sending it out again.

To vary this exercise, imagine that you are breathing any quality in and out of all the pores of your skin—for example, love, compassion, beauty, strength, wisdom, or any quality you desire. Imagine that your breath is a vehicle to receive these attributes and to shine them out into the world to heal yourself and others.

. . . .

EXERCISE: THE CONTINUOUS BREATH

Breathing in and out through your nose, inhale fully, filling your torso with air, and without pausing, exhale fully, expelling all the air from your chest and belly. In the continuous breath, you inhale and exhale fully without pausing on the inhale or the exhale. After several moments of breathing this way, take a deep breath through your mouth, exhale with a sigh, and breathe normally.

. . . .

EXERCISE: THE "AAAHHH" BREATH

Close your eyes and inhale fully, filling your lungs with oxygen, and exhale completely with a sigh. Once more, breathe in, filling your lungs with energy, and now, as you exhale, open your mouth and make the sound "aaaaaaaahhhhhhhh" as you let go of the air fully.

Again, inhale fully, filling your torso with energy, and open your mouth as you exhale, making the sound "aaaaaaaahhhhhhhh," fully and completely, until all the air is released through your lungs.

As you repeat the procedure, close your eyes, and feel the vibration in your body as you expel the air and sustain the sound, "aaaaaaaahhhhhhhh." Place your hand on your chest, solar plexus, and lower belly, directing the sound to the various parts of your body and feeling the resonance. Do this at least ten times. If you have been sitting, lie down and feel the benefit. Open to receive the relaxation.

. . . .

EXERCISE: THE MINDFUL BREATH

In mindful breathing, you sit and become aware of your breath as you inhale and exhale. If thoughts come into your mind, notice them and gently bring yourself back to your breath. Sit for at least ten minutes, simply watching your breath.

This is a wonderful exercise to bring out into your daily life. Begin to watch your breath as you perform simple activities in your life such as driving in your car, fixing a meal, playing golf, sitting at your desk, or taking out the trash. Now watch your breath (and your thoughts) as you interact with others. Notice the temptation to leave your breath and how often you are wanting approval from others, security, or control instead of focusing on your breath. When conversing with others, simply observe yourself and your breath, without trying to change anything.

Bring the movement of your breath into the forefront of your awareness, above anything else that is happening, including your response to other people. You may find that your concentration, your ability to be present, and your relationships all begin to improve. Watch your breath when you are making the decision to eat and while you are actually eating. As your mindfulness increases, notice how your behaviors begin to shift.

. . . .

EXERCISE: THE PANTING BREATH

Begin with a complete inhalation and exhalation. Now begin to pant, focusing on your exhalation and keeping your inhalation brief. Your exhalation should be about twice as long as your inhalation as you pant. You can continue to pant for up to a full minute, breathing through either your nose or your mouth. At the end of a cycle of panting, take a few deep breaths and rest. If you are panting through your mouth, experiment with panting through your nose only.

. . . .

EXERCISE: AFFIRMATIVE BREATHING

Here's a great exercise adopted from the teachings of Vietnamese Buddhist Monk, Thich Nhat Hahn. As you inhale, say to yourself, "I am breathing in." As you exhale, tell yourself, "I am breathing out." Continue this for a cycle of four long, slow, deep breaths. Next, as you inhale, affirm to yourself, "Breathing in, I breathe in peace." As you slowly exhale, tell yourself, "Breathing out, I breathe out peace." On the next breath, "Breathing in, I let go," "Breathing out, I let go." Continue for another cycle of four breaths for each affirmation. As you repeat the phrases with your breath, allow your whole body to sink down, relax, and let go completely of any tension you may be holding.

The Benefits of Regular Practice

As you practice the breathing exercises, pay attention to your body. Take a mental note of how your body feels before the breathing exercise and how you feel after your practice session. If you get dizzy from the exercises, start out slowly and do fewer repetitions. It may take a while for your body to get used to receiving more oxygen.

Be aware of feelings of constriction and expansion in your body. Notice how your breathing changes throughout the day when you take the time to spend a few minutes practicing the breathing exercises daily. I find that even spending five or ten minutes on breathing exercises helps to increase my awareness of my breath throughout the day. It's difficult to breathe in a shallow way consciously. When our awareness increases, the breath deepens naturally. The fuller and deeper your breathing, the more energized and relaxed you are likely to feel. The need for stimulants disappears. Instead, you become filled with and conscious of the life force pumping blood through the veins, keeping you alive.

The more conscious we are of the breath, and the more we breathe down into the belly and pelvis naturally, the more we come in touch with our physical body and the places where we may be holding tension. You may discover that you can no longer wear clothing that is too tight— it's just too uncomfortable, and now you are much more conscious of that than ever before. The comfort of your body becomes a priority.

As you practice the breathing exercises, you may find yourself more aware of tightness in your muscles and places where you may be holding tension. The awareness alone is enough to make huge shifts in the way you carry yourself. Without judging or analyzing, your gentle attention to the places of constriction in your body can help them to simply let go and release. You can even give certain muscles the simple command "Let go. Release," as you breathe into any area that feels tight.

Transitioning from shallow breathing to deep, full belly breathing will help you to sleep better and feel more rested, calmer, and energized, so that you no longer need to turn to food to physiologically change your state. Deep breathing will bring your cells the oxygen they have been crying out for. When you also include physical activity and stretching in your daily regime, along with the breathing, you will find your energy level soaring to new heights.

6. Improve Your Mood and Increase Your Energy with Movement

When you learn to feed your body what it truly requires—much-needed oxygen—via deep breathing and exercise, coupled with high-nutrition foods and a deeper connection to your own heart, you will no longer seek energy ineffectively through the processed, empty-calorie foods that you used to eat. In order to be free from food addiction and unhealthy cravings forever, exercise needs to be a vital component of your daily health regime. It absolutely has to be nonnegotiable, not necessarily just for weight loss, but also for optimum health.

Know that no matter how you feel about exercising on any particular day, when you continue to include movement as part of your daily activity you enhance the overall function of your body and improve your psychological, physiological, and biochemical well-being. This is the state of balance that will help free you from unhealthy cravings and increase your attraction to health-promoting foods.

Physical activity should feel good, and it has enormous benefits. It improves your sleep, increases energy, and decreases stress. Exercise enhances your sense of well-being and improves self-esteem. Regular, consistent exercise also prevents many health problems. It increases bone, heart, and lung strength, decreases blood pressure, and lowers the risk of heart disease and diabetes. It also has the wonderful added benefit of increasing your metabolism so that you are burning more calories, both when you are moving and while you are at rest (including sleeping!).

Approaching Exercise in a New Way

Instead of thinking of exercise as a "should," "must," or painful chore, you can begin to relate to the movement of your body as a pleasant gift that you give to yourself. For example, find some music that you love of any genre—it could be classical, new age, jazz, reggae, or pop. Now turn on the music, adjusting the volume to your liking, and just let your body begin to move—easily, effortlessly, sensually—flowing to the music. There is no right or wrong way to move your body. Simply feel the ecstasy of the movement of your limbs, your arms, your legs, the motion of your torso and head and neck. As you feel your body, also open your awareness to the field of empty space around you that your body is moving through. Close your eyes and melt into the sensation of the dance and the sound of the music, the feel of the beat . . . allow your dance to be erotic or playful, fast or slow . . . remember there is no right or wrong—just the freedom to move . . . to be . . . to breathe fully.

This is what exercise is meant to be in your life—a source of joy, expression, stress-reduction, health, and freedom. The reason exercise may not fit this description for you is because the habits you have developed over time and old programming are standing in your way. You may expect exercise to be painful or something that you have to do to get over with, and certainly not something that brings you a sense of joy and well-being. Part of the reason for this could be that you haven't allowed yourself to find activities that you really love and enjoy. If you don't like riding a bike or swimming, do not choose those as your main form of exercise. Find something that you love to do and are willing to commit to daily.

Back when I was making unhealthy lifestyle choices, I used to love to run. Every day, rain or shine, I would put on my headset and run the three and a half-mile circle in Prospect Park, Brooklyn. This started out as a very positive habit. Soon, however, it became compulsive. I couldn't miss a day, or I would become horribly depressed. If my knee hurt or I was tired one day, I ignored it and ran anyway. So even though exercise is a very healthful activity, I was using it in the wrong way. Running was the mechanism I used to regulate my weight, since my diet was high in simple carbohydrates and sugars.

As I began to use the methods in this book to live a healthier lifestyle, I became aware of how I was using both food and exercise in an unhealthy, compulsive manner. When done in moderation, jogging is a very beneficial, aerobic exercise. However, when it turns into a compulsion that you inflict on yourself as a punishment for overeating, it has the potential to become a form of self-abuse.

The purpose of following the methods of *Easy Sugar Break-Up* is not only to stop consuming foods and liquids that are stimulating an addictive response, but also to develop a much healthier relationship with your body, mind, emotions, and spirit. When you learn to honor your body, activity, deep rest, and healthful eating become a natural result.

Even though I enjoy many forms of activity, including dance, yoga, jumping on a trampoline, bicycling, water exercise, and hiking, for me the best physical regime to commit to is walking.

Walking is something that you can do anywhere, anytime, and in any weather, once you adopt the mindset that this is so. I also love walking because I do most of my movement outside, so I have the added pleasure of fresh air and enjoying various types of scenery. When I walk in the city, watching the people, seeing the buildings, and beating the traffic lights turns my walking into a game.

One hour of walking through a city can feel like five minutes to me as I become caught up in the interesting and diverse surroundings of which I become a part. Walking through the woods gives me a chance to enjoy the beauty and solitude of nature and enhances my connection to the outdoors. Even trudging through the snow on a blustery winter's day gives me a feeling of being alive, as the smell of firewood burning and the comforts of the snowy season flood my senses. When I am home in Florida, I have the thrill of getting up while the rest of my family is in deep slumber and walking on the quiet, still beach, enjoying the sound, smell, and sight of the surf as it laps up onto the hard sand beneath my feet.

Anticipating the Joy of Movement

Is it always easy to get up out of bed and get outside? No, some days it isn't. Nowadays, I take time to listen to my body. If I am really feeling exhausted, then I allow myself the pleasure of a little extra time for slumber and rest. However, on most days it's something that I look forward to. You, too, can look forward to physical activity, when you focus on the benefits, rather than the willpower it's going to require for you to follow through.

For example, when I wake up, I imagine how good it will feel to be outside in the fresh air during my favorite time of day—just before dawn. I imagine that if I wait and try to go out later instead, there may be many obstacles, such as being caught up in the schedule of the day and the needs of other people. Also, I remind myself how special the morning is—so still and quiet, and how expansive the beach will feel, even imagining the gentle breeze against my skin and the feel of my feet pounding on the earth—reveling in the emptiness that characterizes the ocean at that time of day.

Finally, I let myself know that if I am still tired after my morning walk, I can always go back to sleep later, or practice deep relaxation or breathing meditation to get the deep rest that my body needs. I know from experience that physical exercise, deep relaxation, and breathing often gives me more fulfillment and energy than extra sleep. The more we trust and follow what our body really needs, the easier it is to do.

It's also important to tune in to the power of positive momentum. If you choose not to exercise one day, and then you make the same choice the next day, you need to understand that it will most likely be even harder to get motivated on subsequent days because the force of your positive momentum will have been stalled. In the same way, the more we practice destructive behaviors, such as being sedentary or consuming harmful foods or beverages, the greater the likelihood that we will make those same choices again in the future. We are creatures of habit. Maintaining useful routines such as a consistent regime of physical activity and abstaining from harmful actions makes it much more likely that you will continue to repeat the same constructive behaviors. Establishing a positive habit reinforces and strengthens your inner commitment and your deep desire to fulfill the intention you have set for yourself. Success breeds success.

How Can You Stay Motivated?

You may have an aversion to exercise that you need to over-come before you can learn to stay motivated. If you associate exercise with dieting or hard work, it makes sense that you would try to avoid it. These associations may have developed because in the past you only began an exercise regime when you were "on a diet."

If you constantly exercise when you are hungry or not consuming enough calories, it can leave you feeling weak and exhausted, as opposed to energized. It's imperative that you make sure you are eating enough food so that you have the energy to exercise. You should not abuse your body with unrealistic amounts of exercise either. You need to make sure that you're getting enough carbohydrates, albeit complex carbohydrates, in your diet, so that you can burn them as fuel. You'll want to avoid burning protein, which is needed for hormones, bones, and muscles.

You may have avoided exercise because you have an injury or are limited physically in some way. If you find activity difficult to do because of your physical condition, try water exercise. Even people with aches and pains often find that water aerobics, walking in the water, or swimming is easy to do. Yoga and can help heal certain kinds of back pain, although be sure to consult with your doctor if you have an injury and are attempting yoga for the first time.

There can be no more opposition when you consider that exercise is an essential component of your lifestyle today in order to create the kind of tomorrow you are committed to. You may have doubts about your ability to incorporate physical activity into your lifestyle, based on your current self-image. Remember that the past does not equal the future. Rather than dwelling on any negative scenarios from the past, focus on what inspires you to take new, more insightful action in the present. Change is possible if you continue to inquire from within, "What new action can I adopt today that will keep me from repeating mistakes from the past and instead reshape my destiny?"

The key to consistent motivation is your long- and short-term commitment to yourself and your health. If your only incentive is a short-term gain—such as fitting into a certain pair of pants—then your enthusiasm for your chosen activity is likely to be short-lived. Personally, if my only goal were to lose weight, I probably would have lost interest in maintaining an active lifestyle a long time ago.

After all, it's so easy to convince ourselves that we don't really need to exercise. The voice of the self may say, "What's the use? Even if you exercise vigorously for thirty minutes, you're not going to burn enough calories to change your body shape," or "Why subject yourself to the burden of exercise? What difference do a few pounds make anyway?" or "My husband loves me either way, why should I knock myself out?" We can talk ourselves out of exercise no sooner than the idea of getting up off the couch pops into our head.

In order to stay motivated, you have to make exercise appealing and enticing so that you stay committed to regular activity as a way to feel better mentally, emotionally, and physically. The desire to be healthy and fit has to come from the inside. If your regime of physical activity feels like just another set of rules imposed from the outside, it will only trigger rebellion in you. Once again, you need to create within yourself a momentum that is hooked into your own deep inner values and intention in order to create sufficient cause to want to follow through.

To accomplish this, create new, positive rules for yourself that are aligned with your goals. Your rule may be as simple as telling yourself that every morning you will do twenty sit-ups on the edge of your bed, or putting a basket on your bike and committing to riding to the grocery store every afternoon. You may commit to walking for a minimum of thirty minutes, three to five times a week. Create rules that you want to live by because they make sense and support your true desire. Perhaps you have reached the understanding that the only way to truly break long-term, destructive eating tendencies is to create new rules for yourself that include new, positive behaviors. The next very important step is to connect your new rules to the overriding purpose of your life.

Linking Exercise to Your Core Values and Positive Intention

Refer back to the exercise "Connecting with Your Core Values" in Chapter 1 and remind yourself what is important to you. Perhaps it's your relationships, or your self-image as an honest person, or world peace. Whatever you discover your values are, use them to motivate you to begin to care for yourself more deeply.

If your highest value is having fun and being in the moment, then see how viewing exercise as a source of joy and spontaneity makes it more compelling. If your value is to spend time with your children enjoying each other, imagine what a good time you will have Rollerblading with your kids or going for a long bike ride together. Think of the bonding you can do with your family as you swim or dance together. If you discovered in the core values exercise that you deeply value truthfulness, then realize the importance of being honest with yourself when it comes to exercise. If telling yourself that one little cookie won't hurt you or that you'll join the gym next week is a way that you are deceiving yourself, how does that make you feel? Tune in to that feeling to give you the impetus to change your ways, and make your actions reflect the person you aspire to be.

Stepping Into Success

One of the greatest pitfalls to incorporating activity into your lifestyle for good is likely to be letting your weight be your primary goal and your main indicator of success. Let your measurement of accomplishment simply be whether you are moving your body consistently. Congratulate and reward yourself for maintaining an ongoing regime of physical activity, regardless of any other outer benefit you may or may not notice.

Also, don't judge yourself according to unattainable standards. If right now your only exercise is walking to the mailbox and back every day, it's unrealistic to think that you are going to start jogging three miles a day. Instead, you may consider doing five to ten jumping jacks every morning when you get out of bed, along with signing up for a local water exercise class that meets three times a week. Make your goals realistic, and write them down to impress them on your subconscious mind. Better yet, share them with a friend to increase your level of commitment.

It's also very reassuring to know that, like all the other behaviors we engage in (both positive behaviors like brushing our teeth and negative ones like reaching for candy), exercise soon becomes a habit—a very constructive habit. You only have to expend some conscious effort in the very beginning, but after that you'll find the strong impulse to continue with your new chosen behavior welling up from deep inside yourself.

Your only job is to believe that what you want—health and freedom from food addiction forever—is absolutely possible. You need to develop a sense of certainty, which may require a "fake it till you make it" mentality at first. Success hinges on your developing a belief that what you want is possible and beginning to see yourself differently. When you start to act in accordance with your new beliefs, you will be well on your way to claiming your power and the result that you desire in your life.

The Power of Affirmations

We create new beliefs by being willing to change our perceptions. This willingness opens us up to new possibilities beyond what our conscious mind may have thought was possible. Imagery will lock these new thoughts in place. Affirmations and positive imagery are wonderful tools to help you stay motivated to exercise.

An affirmation acts like a magnet to attract to yourself the desired goal. When we repeat statements to ourselves, we start to believe them and act on them. Begin to tell yourself some of the following affirmations throughout the day:

"I love to exercise."

"It feels good to move my body." "My body feels great."

"I am happy to be alive."

"Physical movement energizes me." "I can't wait to run and play." "When I walk, I feel great."

"I radiate optimum health."

"My muscles are firm and strong." "I love myself."

"I take excellent care of myself."

To increase your receptivity to these new ideas, begin to imagine yourself following through on your goals by practicing the following exercise.

. . . .

EXERCISE: THE JOY OF MOVEMENT

Imagine yourself feeling healthy, vibrant, and fit. If there was ever a time when you felt the way you wish to feel—confident, in control of your life and your eating habits, free from addiction—remember that time now. Notice all the details that are present in this image—the sights, textures, and what you are hearing. Use all your senses to make it real for you. Remember any sounds that were present, including what you said to others and what they said to you.

Notice any smells or fragrances in the air. What were you seeing? What were you wearing? Visualize that now—vivid, bright, close, and clear. Go back in time and step into that experience fully. Feel all the pleasurable sensations. Become very associated with that state, meaning that you see the whole scenario through your own eyes, not watching yourself from outside.

Step into that younger you who was fit, energetic, and happy—free from the problem of food cravings and loving physical movement. If there was never such a time, use your imagination and envision that you are healthy, active, and fully alive. Imagine that as you are enjoying a vigorous activity such as dancing, brisk walking, swimming, bicycling, or running, all the systems of your body—your brain, your endocrine and immune systems—are becoming healthier and more balanced.

Anchor this state by giving yourself a phrase to remember that brings back this scenario for you. Tell yourself this phrase now in a very distinctive tone and volume, so you can repeat it later when you wish to retrieve this positive state. You may even imagine some fun, upbeat music behind your statement. Allow this phrase to become an anchor for you—meaning a signal that can bring back this feeling at any point in the future when you wish to recall it. Identify this peak state with your chosen sentence, spoken in a specific tone, in a certain volume. Practice breaking your state of enjoying exercise by thinking of something else or making a brief phone call. Then see if you can bring back your peak state by restating your chosen phrase.

To gain mastery over your ability to recall your peak state at will, you will need to practice it. Throughout the day, take time to imagine yourself exercising and enjoying to the fullest the sensations of moving your body. As you practice the exercise, you may even imagine how good it feels to sweat, to reach an altered state through the movement of your body. Imagine your adrenals releasing spirit-lifting chemicals of happiness such as norepinephrine and encephalin. Studies have shown that these natural chemicals help to eliminate depression and induce the "runner's high" you may have heard about or experienced.

Imagery and affirmations are a powerful way to effect desired changes in your perceptions of both exercise and your food preferences. Remember that your subconscious mind is just a blank computer that accepts any programming.

When you imagine yourself in peak states of energy and joy, your heart and lungs filling with oxygen, your limbs pumping to the beat of some upbeat music, you begin to program your mind to want to follow through on these actions. The more detailed you make the imagery—even imagining the exact sequence of events using all your senses—the more your new programming will take root in the recesses of your mind and lead to a new reality for you.

Thought always precedes action, so by changing your thoughts to reflect your deepest intention to live a more fulfilling life, you can begin to reshape your life and your destiny. Internally, you can change what certain behaviors represent to you. In the past, physical movement may have conjured up images of sore muscles and exhaustion. As you work to reframe those images, activity can begin to symbolize freedom, well-being, and a new way of life.

Combining Breathing with Movement

When you stretch your muscles while taking deep, full breaths, you are sending energy-giving oxygen to vital parts of your body. Also, breathing into and stretching your muscles increases your energy level naturally.

. . . .

EXERCISE: THE MORNING STRETCH

An invigorating way to wake up and energize yourself is to stand up with your arms at your sides, your feet hip-width apart. Now inhale fully as you lift your arms up to the sky. As you exhale forcefully through your mouth, bend forward at the waist and, with your knees very slightly bent, let your hands touch the floor (or as far as they can go), holding your breath out for a moment. As you come up again, once more lift your arms up high as you inhale, hold your breath for a moment, and then exhale forcefully through your mouth as you once more bend at the waist, relaxing your knees slightly and letting your arms and hands hang down.

A variation of this exercise is to lift your arms up to the ceiling and then bend forward at the waist, allowing your hands and arms to hang down toward the floor. In this bent-over position, inhale and exhale fully several times, allowing each breath to fill your lungs even more completely. Imagine the breath filling your whole torso all the way down into your pelvis as your muscles relax more and more. You can hold this pose for a few moments and, when you are ready, come up to a standing position. Arch your back slightly and bring your arms overhead to achieve the opposite stretch in your chest and abdominal muscles.

I highly recommend that you take a local stretching, Pilates, or yoga class, which combine breathing and movement to help you get attuned to your body. Yoga is a wonderful choice because breath is such an integral part of the poses.

Breathing into and stretching your muscles removes toxic buildup in the muscle tissues. Once you learn some stretches in a formal class, it becomes much easier to incorporate stretching into your daily life. Throughout the day, you may find moments when you can slip into and hold a runner's pose, or do some shoulder lifts by raising your shoulders up to your ears. Slow and gentle head and neck rolls can be a great way to relieve tension. Perhaps you'll find yourself getting down on the floor, spreading out your legs, and touching your toes. One of my favorite ways to bring relief to my body is to roll on the floor, with my knees up to my chest and my arms hugging my knees, giving my spine a nice massage. The possibilities are enormous, once stretching and breathing become a part of your conscious awareness and daily repertoire of health-promoting activities.

Look Forward to Unexpected Benefits

It doesn't matter which form of exercise you choose, only that you consistently move your body in order to reap tremendous health benefits. By far, the greatest perk of an increased activity level is the improvement in the quality of your life. Aside from curbing cravings, your new regime will leave you with a much calmer and happier state of mind and an increase in physical energy and self-confidence. Also movement, as you will discover, plays a vital role in the Break-Your-Craving-State Technique by allowing you to let go of old, unwanted emotions and patterns from the past much more quickly. Let's take a look, in the next chapter, at the powerful technique that can help you change your state from feeling out of control with food cravings to feeling strong, empowered, and in control of your life and your eating habits.

7. The Break-Your-Craving-State Technique

Though it's impossible to force yourself to not think about something (try to not think about a pink elephant), you can certainly change the lens through which you are looking at something. We can take our focus away from the limited mind (negative chatter) and instead perceive ourselves and our lives through the lens of the heart. Now that you know how to identify your emotional and physical needs (are you truly hungry—or are you thirsty or tired?) and give yourself love and are familiar with deep breathing exercises and the incredible benefit of movement, you are ready for the Break-Your-Craving-State Technique.

When we enter a state of having intense food cravings, it is often because we are reacting to a particular trigger, such as an uncomfortable or disturbing interaction or the occurrence of a stressful event. We then go into a stressed state—perhaps our muscles in the belly, jaw, shoulders, or pelvis become clenched unconsciously or we find ourselves feeling numb or agitated.

Habitually, this state can then be accompanied by an intense craving for certain foods—often the foods that we think of as comforting. Until we find a way to break this inner state, we remain a slave to the triggers in our environment. Also, we often use food or drugs habitually as an efficient means to change our state—that is, to change the way that we are feeling in the moment. If you're like many of my clients, your unproductive eating habits have developed and been reinforced for many years.

The Break-Your-Craving-State Technique offers you a method for breaking the internal state that causes your cravings without having to self-medicate with food, alcohol, caffeine, drugs—both prescription and otherwise, or diet pills, and it teaches you how to move from your outer level—where your doubts and fears about yourself and your environment exist—to the deeper levels inside yourself where the states of being that free you from addiction reside.

Breaking Free from Habitual Responses

Before you can effectively break your state, you need to acknowledge the state that you are in. Many times when we are "out of sorts," we are unclear as to what is really happening internally. Often it appears as if we were simply responding to outside circumstances. For example, we may tell ourselves, "Of course I am upset and reaching for the candy jar—my son has been screaming for half an hour," or "It's no wonder I'm going to need to drink a pot of coffee today—I was up all night with the dog," or "I was treated so poorly as a child, I'll always seek to comfort myself with chips and bread."

These statements seem self-evident. However, if your goal is to live your life healthfully and happily and care for and honor your body, heart, and mind, then reaching for the candy jar or chips or drinking the pot of coffee is in conflict with the intention that you set. Project ahead and ask yourself, how are you going to feel after you engage in the behavior? Even if the candy distracts you from the upset with your son, or the bread gives you a few moments of relief from unpleasant feelings, or the coffee helps you to get through the day, you are very likely to feel remorseful and bad about yourself, and may even come to the conclusion that you are hopeless.

One of the difficulties with changing our inner state is that our automatic patterns of reacting to life become ingrained on our nervous system. Also, we often don't believe that we are worthy of trading in our painful condition for a newer, happier reality.

So even though there is an infinite number of possible choices each of us could make in any given moment, we tend to repeat the same patterns—and experience similar results— even when the outer situation is different. For example, if you tend to experience a state of feeling overwhelmed, it is likely that this state will reoccur even if your circumstances change. You may feel overwhelmed when you are at work because of your heavy workload and the unreasonable deadlines that are placed on you. However, when you quit your job, to your dismay, you may experience the exact same feeling—but now it may be in relationship to how much effort it takes to keep your house clean. Your response to this state of feeling overwhelmed—bingeing or being sedentary—may be the same in both situations. This is why Band-Aid approaches like going on a diet rarely work over the long haul. In order to see lasting change, you need to get to the root of the issue and clear and heal it.

What if there was a way to break your state in such situations, rather than follow the familiar road of self-sabotage? Wouldn't it be wonderful to change your course midstream and switch to the path that leads you to your desired destination? The Break-Your-Craving-State Technique will allow you to do just that.

Let's take a look at some of the underlying states that lead to food addiction or addiction in general as well as those internal states that can free you from persistent food and substance cravings.

Inner States That Lead to Food Addiction

- Confused

- Nervous

- Afraid

- Anxious

- Perplexed

- Weak

- Sad

- Depressed

- Ashamed

- Manic

- Excited

- Worried

- Unsafe

- Threatened

- Judged

- Out of control

- Lonely

- Frustrated

- Hopeless

- Desperate

- Insecure

- Powerless

Inner States That Free You from Food Addiction

- Joy

- Bliss

- Peace

- Calm

- Tranquility

- Strength

- Hope

- Love

- Connection

- Happiness

- Fulfillment

- Aliveness

- Safety

- Acceptance

- Protection

- Patience

- Gratitude

- Fullness

The Method

The following seven-step Break-Your-Craving-State Technique is to be used any time you experience unhealthy cravings. During the two weeks of your Mega-Nutrition Cleanse (see Chapter 11), I recommend that you practice this exercise every day. This will help you to release your attachment to many of your emotional triggers around food, at the same time that your body is being cleansed of your physical addictions to certain foods.

To practice this exercise effectively, activate your imagination. As you repeat the practice daily, there will be many sessions when you aren't actually triggered, in the moment, when you are going through this exercise. For those times, I recommend that you imagine your last negative eating experience or substance binge and recall the triggers and internal state that you were in.

This type of practice will make it easier to employ the technique when you are actually in a situation where you need it. Also, some of the steps require time and privacy. Therefore, the more you practice the technique in a quiet and private place while imagining your food triggers, the easier it will be to use it in a more charged situation when you are actually caught in the throes of food, alcohol or drug cravings.

The Break-Your-Craving-State Technique

1. Distance yourself from the trigger.

2. Identify your inner state.

3. Get a second, truer opinion.

4. Identify with your new state.

5. Shake off the limiting belief.

6. Anchor your higher intention.

7. Choose a new action.

Step 1: Distance Yourself from the Trigger

The first step of the Break-Your-Craving-State Technique is to notice that you are about to overeat, binge, eat the wrong foods, or engage in any addictive, unproductive behavior around food, or any other substance. As soon as you have that realization, *stop*. Give yourself some mental space: literally become aware of the space that surrounds you and the space that your body occupies. Allow your focus to switch from your thinking mind (between your ears) to the vast spaciousness that you are. When we enter a craving state, we often narrow our focus to include only a particular set of thoughts, feelings, and images associated with our craving. The purpose of giving yourself this mental space is to expand your awareness beyond the immediate trigger. Breathe into the space within and around you, become aware of the sights and smells and sounds of the room you are in, as well as the emptiness around the objects and the silence out of which all sounds emerge.

Step 2: Identify Your Inner State

Next, turn your attention back to your thoughts. Notice what your dominant thoughts are, as you did in Chapter 4, and begin to write them down, if you are able.

"I can't take it anymore." "He's driving me crazy."

"I must be a really bad mother." "This sucks."

"I need a cookie."

"I shouldn't have one."

"My stomach is in a knot."

"That's it—I'm just going to turn on the TV and eat some chips."

"My nerves are shot. I need to take a pill."

"It's almost 5pm. I can have a drink."

"I'll always be fat. I can't stick to anything."

Based on these internal voices, name your current state. If you can't narrow it down to one on the list of inner states that lead to food addiction, choose several or create your own. Perhaps the state you would identify yourself to be in would be anxiety, self-judgment, and emotional pain.

Now go down your list of voices and see if there is any one voice that sums up this feeling. It's OK if you can't discern one or two voices—you can do the next part of the method on as many voices as you need to. But let's say that as you look at your list of voices, you realize that the main theme is "My life is out of control," and perhaps the additional judging voice that says, "It shouldn't be this way."

Notice how your body feels when you listen to these negative voices. It is important, while you are on Step 2, to have complete acceptance of your thoughts and feelings without judging them. Interestingly, the more you judge yourself, the more you keep the very conditions in place that you wish to change.

Therefore, it's necessary to give yourself space while you are in this challenging state. Accept your inner state, even though it's not your preference. Just as fighting with the weather won't change it, opposing your inner reality won't make it different. Only by giving yourself acceptance, understanding, and compassion can you grow into the person that you aspire to be. Criticism and judgment, especially from within yourself, only hinders the process.

Step 3: Get a Second, Truer Opinion

The next step is to question the validity of these internal voices. To do that, take a moment and imagine that your deep inner wisdom could speak. You connect to your deeper wisdom through your heart. Place your hand on your heart, bow your head to your chest, and breathe into the center of your chest—your deep, metaphorical heart. When you place your hand on the center of your upper chest (as opposed to the left side of your chest where your physical heart is) and breathe into that area, you can get in touch with a very subtle place that I call the soft heart.

It's a place of softness, tenderness, openness, and loving-kindness that you can tap into and take refuge in by making the conscious choice to focus on it and open your feeling awareness. When you are in touch with the soft spot in your heart, ask your inner wisdom for guidance by inquiring within, "If my higher self or inner wisdom could speak, what would it say about that negative voice?"

It may be helpful for you to personify your deeper wisdom by imagining that it is coming to you from a real or fictitious teacher, one of your beloved, wise ancestors, a dear friend, or perhaps a prophet or angel whom you trust, love, and respect.

For example, what would a dear friend say in response to the voices telling you that you are overweight, a helpless addict and undeserving of love? What would an angel say to you at a time when you feel so angry, hurt, or alone? Write down any response that you get. If you don't get anything, simply write down the opposite thought. If your original thought was "I'm pathetic," write down the opposite, "I am strong and beautiful." Do not worry if your conscious mind thinks it's a true statement. At the deepest level, your first voice is not true either.

Look at the phrases that sum up your state that you wrote down on your paper—"My life is out of control" and "It shouldn't be this way," and ask your friend, esteemed ancestor, angel, beloved prophet, or higher self to give you his or her perspective. Take as much time as you need, however, the process should be effortless.

If it feels in any way effortful, simply skip that part and write down the opposite thought. If your original thoughts were "It shouldn't be this way. I feel weak. I am out of control," your opposite thoughts may be "My life is happening perfectly, according to a bigger plan that I don't know about. I am stronger than I feel." You may also add, "I am in control of my life and my eating habits."

Step 4: Identify with Your New State

The next step is to ask yourself, "If these new thoughts, given to me by my higher self, Divine Love or wise teacher, were true, what would my state be?" Take a look at the list of states of being that free you from addiction found earlier in this chapter, and choose one or more that resonate for you now. To help you, keep repeating these new phrases silently or out loud until you feel the impact of their meaning on your heart, for example, "Wow, it's true—I really am in control of my life and my eating habits. My life is perfect exactly as it is. I accept that."

Breathe in the new statement and feel what your new state would be if that were true. If a voice pops in telling you that it's not true, just disregard it. Send that destructive voice off. It's just testing you. If evidence of your negative state creeps in, recognize that this is based on your past.

What is your new, positive state? Write that state down. Use any image that you can to make this state real for you and embed it into the cells of your body. Use all your senses. This will help you to relax both physically and mentally and release you from the grip of your previous negative state. There are many possible ways for you to do this, so find the one that works for you.

One way would be for you to use all your senses and see, feel, smell, taste, and hear a magnificent, bright or colorful, fresh waterfall that embodies your state emanating from above your head. For example, if your state is safety and gratitude, you can even imagine this waterfall of safety and gratitude flowing into your body and filling every bone, every muscle, every cell and fiber of your being. You can then take your visualization a step further by feeling this waterfall of magnificent higher qualities flowing through you and into the earth below your feet—grounding you and connecting you from the heavens to the earth. You may see the words *safety* and *gratitude* written in light above your head or in your heart. The more real you can make the image, the greater the benefit you will receive, and the stronger the impact this new state will have on you.

Stand or sit in the waterfall of safety and gratitude (in this case) until you really feel a shift inside yourself. This shift may be a relaxation of your muscles, a deepening of your breathing, a heaviness or lightness in your limbs, a tingling sensation in your fingers or toes, or simply a sense of openness and expansion. When that feels solid you can put your thumb and your forefinger together as you repeat your phrase in order to anchor in this new way of being in the world. A kinesthetic anchor such as putting your two fingers together while you repeat your affirmative word or phrase is a way to make your resourceful state easier to access throughout the day, when you need it most.

It's essential that you become grounded in this new state because right now you are in a precarious position—caught between two possible states. Depending on which one you ultimately choose, you will experience a very remarkable and distinct difference in your life. So the next few steps are going to stack the odds in favor of you selecting the state that will lead you to the life that you desire and deserve.

Step 5: Shake Off the Limiting Belief

Part of this process requires breaking the old patterns. It's very helpful to realize that lowering the intensity of your difficult emotions can be a cumulative process. Therefore, it is beneficial to go back to the original negative state that resulted from being triggered in order to insure that you aren't simply repressing the emotion, but truly letting it go and healing any old wounds that got stirred up. To help you recall your original triggered state, go back and look at your first few statements—the ones you wrote down when you were in a state of anxiety and self-judgment.

To help diffuse the feelings of the challenging state that was triggered in you, you are going to use breath, sound, and movement, since these methods can have a very dramatic effect on your state of being. You can take any of the breathing exercises that you learned in Chapter 5 and use them in combination with movement that you feel comfortable with. Filling your body with oxygen and changing your physiology are ways to physically break your attachment to your earlier state of negativity. You may just want to shake your arms and legs vigorously and let your whole body express itself by moving.

A playful alternative is to imagine that you are an animal and make the movements and sounds of this animal. This will help to free you from your identity and help you see the absurdity of dwelling on the negative thoughts as well as their impact on your life. Also, by physically changing your posture, you are automatically breaking your state. Imagine that you are a monkey—scratch your belly and underarms and hop from place to place. Imagine that you are a lion and roar, stretching your lips, tongue, and mouth and jaw muscles.

The more you are able to use sound, breath, and exaggerated movement to shake off your previous state, the better. Open your mouth wide and sigh audibly and fully. Create sound by chanting the vowels of the alphabet, elongating each syllable. Feel the vibration within yourself. Notice how the different sounds that you chant are likely to bring vibration to various parts of your body. For example the short "aaaaah" sound will probably create a resonance in your heart, whereas the "eeeeee" sound may vibrate in your head. As you play with sound and movement, and especially breath, notice how your state begins to shift naturally.

If you're in a public situation, even taking a few deep, full breaths coupled with a subtle stretch of your arms and legs can help you to physically break your state. What you're doing is changing your physiology. By doing so, your psychological state naturally shifts. For example, notice how when you're depressed you tend to look down and slump your shoulders, and when you are happy, you are likely to smile. Our physiology naturally reflects how we feel. Therefore, to help yourself move from a triggered state of being to a more resourceful state, it can be very helpful to change your physiology by altering your breathing, facial expression, and posture and, most important, moving your body!

Step 6: Anchor Your Higher Intention

When you are finished shaking off your negative state through breath, sound, and movement, go back to the image of safety and gratitude (or whatever state had come to you). Now, anchor in your new state even more by putting your two fingers together and repeating your empowering phrase, such as the words *safety* and *gratitude* or "I am safe." Now reset your intention. To do that, place your hand on your heart, close your eyes, and with your breath travel inward behind your outer self as you learned to do in Chapter 1. Imagine a bright, golden, radiant light emanating from the center of your chest, deep inside yourself. Stay with your intention for as long as you need to so you really feel it begin to solidify. Anchor in your intention with your word or phrase. For example, if your intention is to love yourself no matter what the circumstance, you may add to your earlier phrase "I am safe. Only love is real. My heart is filled with love." Allow that intention and phrase to permeate and fill all the levels of your heart. This is your truth. This is your statement to yourself and to the world.

Next, go back to any image that helps you to lock in your new, empowered state, and keeping your hand on your heart and using breath, travel to your deeper layers. Take your time and allow yourself to pass through a portal to the greater spaces within, going deeper and deeper.

When you have reached a silent, spacious place, connect your heart center to your belly with an invisible cord or line of light. Allow this light to flow down into the center of the earth, grounding you. Imagine roots coming out of your legs and feet and grounding you to the earth. As you connect with your belly, allow it to relax and soften completely. Placing one hand on your heart center and one on your belly, reaffirm your true intention to care for and honor yourself, your precious life, and your body—your holy temple—and to only choose actions that are in alignment with your sincere longing. Repeat any word or phrase that assists you in solidifying your intention. To make your new anchor most valuable, it can be helpful to summarize your phrase into one or two words that can most effectively bring back your resourceful state. (For this step, it would be best to read through it first and then repeat it with your eyes closed.)

Step 7: Choose a New Action

Allow your actions to reflect your intention. Imagine yourself acting only in accordance with your highest value— reflecting your commitment to yourself and the freedom you are choosing. Now go back to the situation in your outer life that triggered you originally, and imagine that even with this outer situation happening exactly as it is, you can still maintain your new, more empowered state. Congratulations on your commitment to yourself and your life and the fulfillment of your dreams! In this case, despite the fact that your son is acting out today, you can choose to get through this difficult time without using food as a coping mechanism. Instead, you can connect with your own strength, patience, and self-love.

How to Break Your Craving State When You Are Out in the World

Again, the more you practice this technique at home in response to specific triggers and uncomfortable states that you have experienced, the easier it will be to translate your gains moment-to-moment in situations that come up for you.

For example, the stronger your kinesthetic anchor (putting your thumb and your forefinger together as you repeat a phrase that gives you strength and confidence), the greater the impact it will have on you, and the more effectively it will transform your state into a resourceful one. If you are in a public situation and you are triggered by an event and find yourself feeling weak or powerless, you will be able to fire your anchor (touch your two fingers together) and instantly shift into a peak state of strength and courage. If you feel that there is still some emotional residue from the trigger, later, when you are in the privacy of your home, you can practice the seven-step Break-Your-Craving-State Technique and use the new trigger that came up for you as material.

Repeating the full process over and over is a very powerful

way to gain mastery over the emotional states that in the past led you to food cravings and unproductive behaviors. Soon you will find yourself responding to old situations in a completely fresh way, and positive actions will become a new habit. Going through the seven steps systematically helps you to gain perspective on the event that triggered you, but even more important, it gives you the opportunity to release your old pattern and resolve the feelings rather than simply covering them over. The more you practice anchoring in the positive state, the greater your ability to use that anchor when you are in difficult situations. Even slight changes in your physiology, such as taking a couple of deep breaths, closing your eyes for a moment, or placing your hand on your chest, will help you to find your inner strength when you need it most.

Do You Believe That You Overeat When You Are Happy?

Often my clients will say to me, "I am just as likely to eat when I am happy as when I am upset," or "I have a very happy life, so why would I want to change my state?" These are excellent observations. What I have noticed is that many times we are not really aware of our complete underlying state. If we examine the situation more closely, we may realize that even though we are eating when we are happy or as a way of celebrating, underneath the festivity of the occasion we may have other feelings lurking. So, for example, you may be at a social engagement, and consciously you are having the time of your life.

There are lots of fun people to talk to—you may even be considered the life of the party. In such situations, I urge you to check in and notice how you are feeling underneath the exterior of happiness. Are you feeling nervous or anxious? Even excitement is a state that can have your body keyed up and blocked from true happiness. Are you experiencing any physical tightness in your belly, pelvis, or jaw? Without any judgment, just notice what is really going on for you when you are in that situation.

Unfortunately, we can be habitually unconscious of our true feelings. It is only when we start to practice a technique for conscious relaxation and expansion, such as meditation or self-hypnosis, that we often discover that our natural, every-day state of awareness is far from relaxed or happy in the true sense of the word. Yes, we may be cheerful and enjoying our lives, but if there is an undercurrent of anxiety, fear, or worry, then we are depriving ourselves of true happiness—which I define as a state of bliss, love, peace, unity, and freedom—free from any angst. The anxiety we are so comfortable with could be obvious, but it's just as likely to be completely out of our awareness—until all of a sudden we experience the onset of a migraine, diarrhea, or high blood pressure.

Many of us have learned to internalize our emotions and put a smile on our face. While this may have made you popular, it isn't necessarily the way you want to live for the rest of your life. It's important to admit to yourself what you are truly feeling, because it's only what you feel that you can heal. It's true that our feelings are like the weather—they come and go, without giving us much choice. However, the more we identify with a particular set of thoughts and feelings, the more we create an inner climate maintaining a certain state. As you learned previously, distinct states, such as anxiety or boredom, are likely to result in predictable behaviors, such as eating the wrong foods, or reaching for harmful substances.

If you are in denial either consciously or unconsciously of the states that you experience regularly and the voices and emotions that lead you there, how can you learn from them and experience the gifts that await you when you have the courage to move through these unpleasant states?

Moving through means traveling behind what's apparent or going beyond the limitations of our conscious interpretation of events. On the outer level, you may be aware of anxiety. As you sit with the tension and open to it, you may experience a feeling of being unsafe. When you ask yourself what you're afraid of, you may become aware that you doubt that your needs will be met. Inquiring as to what the remedy is, from your higher, wiser self, you may find that the medicine is patience and trust. Becoming conscious gives you new choices. It's not necessarily easy, but it is essential if you want to break those patterns that are holding you back from living your life happy, healthy, fit, and free from food or any other addiction.

One reason we may have the tendency to hide our true feelings even from ourselves is because we are afraid of the ridicule or shame that may result from our vulnerability. That's why it's so important, as you embark on this journey of healing your overweight or unhealthy condition, that you make a commitment to be really gentle and caring with yourself.

You need to be able to confide in yourself and say, "Right now I am feeling jealous. Typically I would go off by myself and gorge on food. Instead I am just going to go through the Break-Your-Craving-State Technique to take the edge off, see what I learn about myself, and make a better choice."

If you can take a ten-minute break by yourself, that's great, but if that's not possible, don't despair. As you practice at home regularly using your typical triggers, in your imagination, you will soon find that you can employ an abbreviated Break-Your-State easily, even when you are in a public situation. In these difficult circumstances, you must commit to being extremely supportive and compassionate with yourself if you are to turn your life around and change deep-seated behavior patterns. When you can foster an atmosphere of trust within yourself, you'll become more comfortable as you go through both the easy times and the more challenging situations.

Exaggerating Your State

One alternative and effective way to break your current state quickly is to simply exaggerate it to the point of becoming absurd. For example, when you are faced with a situation that brings up painful feelings in you, rather than rationalize or deny your feelings (which often leads to stuffing your feelings with food), you can take the situation to a ridiculous conclusion. I find the following exercise to be extremely helpful in letting go of any attachment to things being a certain way and returning to a state of equilibrium and peace. You'll still have preferences, but wouldn't it be wonderful to be free from the angst that often occurs when people or situations in life inevitably let you down?

Here's how it works. The first step to exaggerating your state is to realize and admit to yourself that you are triggered. It doesn't matter if the trigger is mild or strong. Just notice your physical state. Let's start with the following example, and then you can try it for yourself.

You are feeling slightly annoyed that your friend didn't return your phone call for over a week. Write down (or become aware of) the inner voices:

"Why doesn't she call me back? Doesn't she care about me?"

"She's too busy for our friendship. I really miss her."

"Maybe I should call her again. No, I don't want to bother her."

"I'm just going to forget about her and get busy.

She's always too preoccupied."

"I'm tired of this being a one-way friendship."

Notice how your body feels, and tune in to where in your body you may be holding this feeling of annoyance. Name the predominant feeling. Be honest with yourself. You may write down, "Right now I am feeling really angry with Jane. She never calls me back. I'm busy, too, but I always make time for her. I'm tired of being the one who has to reach out."

Now exaggerate your anger to the point of a ridiculous conclusion. If you followed your anger, uncensored, and allowed it to lead you, where might you end up? Have fun with your scenario. There may be a few options. One may be that Jane finally does call you and you hang up on her. You may imagine that your anger gets so strong that you start yelling and screaming and punching the walls. You may pound so hard on the walls that your house starts to crumble.

By taking the conclusion to the absurd, it's easier to let the feelings flow through you and disappear naturally, without trying to make them go away or acting them out in a self-destructive way. When you exaggerate your state, use all your senses. Increase the accompanying inner voices' rate of chatter. Then slow it down. You may even change the pitch and tempo of your self-talk to make it more ridiculous. If there is a certain person (or yourself) whom you believe is the cause of your upset, see his or her face (or your own) and the entire situation in a very distorted way.

Perhaps as you sit with your anger, you realize that there is some deep sadness underneath. You may discover voices like this underneath:

"I'm all alone."

"All my friends are gone."

"My children grew up so fast."

"Life is lonely."

"I don't have the energy for friendship."

"People always hurt me."

Now, rather than convince yourself that these thoughts are silly and you should get rid of them, once again exaggerate the feelings that these thoughts lead to, and watch them vanish naturally. Notice how you are feeling physically, and once again write down your state: sad, depressed, hopeless, lonely.

Making your states stronger temporarily, and taking the possible outcomes of acting out your feelings to a ridiculous conclusion, helps to loosen their grip on you. The goal is to realize that you do have control over how long and often this scenario gets replayed in your mind's eye. Once you can accept that your internal states come and go it becomes easier to just say yes to what you are feeling in the moment. When you exaggerate that feeling to a very illogical, absurd conclusion, it becomes easier to give up the need to control life, since it is impossible to do so. We come to realize and accept that part of being alive is experiencing all the highs and lows—including joy and sadness, feelings of connection and separation, gains and losses, thrills and disappointments.

An enlightening question to ask yourself is, "How long am I going to hold on to this?" When you realize that you are going to have to let the matter go at some point, it becomes easier to let it go sooner rather than later, especially when you make the connection between holding on to the feelings and judgments and the suffering that you are creating for yourself as a result.

Sometimes it feels convenient or accurate to assume that if a certain situation or person weren't there, you could truly be happy. You may imagine that if only you weren't over-weight, your life would be good. But the truth is that your overweight or unhealthy condition is an opportunity that life is giving you to know and love yourself more deeply. If we view all the challenges in our lives this way, we come to see that every obstacle is a doorway to uncover the greater vir-tues that lie hidden within. The following is a great exercise to use when you are already triggered and need to reach a more resourceful state quickly. Here are the steps:

. . . .

EXERCISE: EXAGGERATE-YOUR-STATE TECHNIQUE

1. Realize that you are triggered.

2. Become aware of the inner voices. Notice how your body feels. If you can, write down the thoughts and feelings on paper.

3. See the situation that is upsetting you in your mind's eye.

4. Exaggerate it in any way that you can. Imagine it much worse than it actually is. Intensify your neg-ative reaction to the people and events that are involved. Bring it to a ridiculous conclusion.

5. Open your heart to yourself and unlock the well of love and compassion that is available from yourself

to yourself. Bring in the images and colors that soothe you. Imagine yourself resting on top of a rainbow, infused by all the healing colors, the illuminating, radiant light washing away any pain or suffering. Imagine a guardian angel or a highly evolved being of divine love holding you and showering you with appreciation and compassion, whispering words of encouragement, adoration, and hope to you.

By practicing both the Break-Your-Craving-State and the Exaggerate-Your-State techniques on a regular basis, you will begin to have more control over your habitual emotional reactions that lead you to crave and eat the wrong foods or put toxic substances into your body. As you clear your old patterns of responding to life, it will get easier and easier to choose healthy foods and a healthier lifestyle. Aside from any emotional causes for food cravings, it is very likely that there is a strong physical component compelling you to reach for foods that perpetuate problems for you. In the next four chapters, "High-Nutrition Eating," "The Truth about CBD," "Sugar Cancelling Recipes," and "The Two-Week Mega-Nutrition Cleanse," you'll learn how to eliminate these physiological yearnings for the wrong foods, how to use a powerful plant cannabinoid-herb to change your mind-body-state, and how to find yourself naturally reaching for those delicious, healthier foods that will keep you craving-free.

Part 3. Eat Smart for Life

8. High-Nutrition Eating

What is high-nutrition eating? It is choosing the foods from the earth, in their most whole and natural state, organic wherever possible, that will sustain you and bring you health. When you are in the habit of grabbing fast food on the go or eating a lot of packaged, processed food, you may not even be aware of other dietary choices and how much better you would feel if your diet consisted of healthy, nutritious, water-rich foods, eaten in balance with healthy fat, complex carbs and pure protein. We take for granted all the highly processed garbage, filled with huge amounts of sugar, fat, chemicals and salt, that we are surrounded by. Foods that are poisonous to our system have become the norm by a vast segment of society. The person who chooses fresh salads and vegetables over canned or frozen meals is often considered a health nut.

If you are going to live your life filled with energy, health, and natural vitality and at your ideal weight, it may be necessary to change your entire thinking about food. Before you get nervous, please be reassured that it is actually very easy. Once you start to eat high-nutrition foods regularly, and preparing them so they taste great, you will never go back to eating the old way, dulling all your senses and slowly poisoning yourself.

High-nutrition eating simply means choosing foods that are natural, unprocessed, whole and from the earth. Foods from the earth are high in vitamins, minerals, fiber, and water. These are the building blocks that your body needs to maintain health and vitality.

What Are Healthy Foods?

Before we look at the foods that may be causing you harm, let's look at the wonderful assortment of foods that bring you health.

Water-Rich Foods

At the top of the list are water-rich foods. This means salads, vegetables, and fruits. The secret to wanting these foods is in the preparation and the combinations of food that you use. Once you learn how to make salads and vegetables taste delicious, you'll no longer have to force yourself to eat them. You'll begin to enjoy them above all other foods and actually miss them when your circumstances don't allow you to choose them. How can you prepare salads and vegetables so they taste good? The key is to eat them with a balance of other nutritious foods so that you feel satisfied. This means combining your salads and vegetables with healthy fats, protein, and complex carbohydrates. These combinations will satisfy you, create a feeling of fullness in your stomach, and supply a steady source of energy to your brain, especially when you are committed to staying away from sugar and simple, processed, refined carbohydrates.

Choose a variety of vegetables including the following:

- Kale

- Collards

- Broccoli

- Cauliflower

- Yellow squash

- Zucchini

- Snow peas

- Red or green cabbage

- Red chard

- Red or green peppers

- Cucumbers

- Leeks

- Onions

- Eggplant

- Tomatoes

- Romaine, leafy green, red, or butter lettuce

- Spring mix

- Bok choy

- Carrots

- Celery

- Beets

Try to vary your vegetables. Select from an array of different colored vegetables for visual delight as well as the full spectrum of vitamins and minerals available from the various plant foods.

Aside from the abundance of phytonutrients that vegetables provide, they are also a wonderful source of fiber. Fiber slows the rate in which food enters your bloodstream. When you include fiber with your meals, you slow down the digestion rate of the entire meal, thus delaying the absorption of sugar and fat and decreasing the need for insulin to be secreted. This eliminates spikes and drops in blood sugar that can wreak havoc on your system and ultimately cause cravings and hunger.

If you like raw veggies, spend a little time cutting them up into tiny pieces. Put them in a plastic container in your refrigerator so they stay fresh for a few days. Then, when you are ready to eat them, combine the vegetables with fresh dark-green lettuce and sprinkle them with cold-pressed olive oil and herbs and perhaps a little sea salt. These types of salads are delicious!

If you prefer your vegetables cooked, take any of the listed vegetables such as cabbage, bok choy, broccoli, or collards, steam them lightly, and then sauté in olive oil with leeks and garlic. You can add a hint of sea salt (available at the health food store).

Eggplant, zucchini, and yellow squash are delicious simply drizzled with olive oil and roasted or broiled in the oven. Do not overcook! Nothing is worse than soggy vegetables. Cooking lightly will help to retain the phytochemicals and other nutrients in the foods, as well as their delicious natural flavors. To make a meal, simply combine the raw or cooked vegetables with animal protein and complex carbohydrate.

If you know that you'll probably need to snack during the day, start carrying around with you little bags of cut-up vegetables such as carrot sticks, celery, fennel (anise), or cucumbers. Diced vegetables with a few raw almonds or a small container with almond butter, are a wonderful snack to keep on hand for hunger "emergencies." You may also need to carry around a small cooler bag with some emergency brain food such as hard-boiled eggs or a small piece of meat (hormone-free, anti-biotic free).

Protein

Protein is also a critical part of a healthy diet. In selecting protein sources, consider the following (preferably organic and hormone-free):

- Lamb

- Beef

- Eggs

- Chicken

- Turkey

- Fish (all types, including tuna, salmon, flounder, grouper, trout, sole, bass, halibut, and others)

To normalize our blood sugar, many of us need to incorporate animal protein into our diet. In fact, if you have symptoms of low blood sugar—mood swings, fatigue, big fluctuations in energy level, jitteriness, strong emotional reactions, or even dizziness, or if you are overweight— chances are you could benefit from making animal protein a mainstay of your diet. Even if you don't like the idea of it, it's very likely that altering your diet by increasing the amount of protein and the frequency with which you eat it would bring you the level of health and freedom from addiction that you are seeking.

Why animal protein? Think about the foods you crave. It is highly unlikely that you crave animal protein in an unhealthy way. It is very difficult to binge on chicken, fish, or meat—unless, of course, it is cooked with or covered in some rich, creamy, oily, salty, or sugary sauce. But protein alone does not cause cravings. In fact, it ends them. Why? Because it satisfies us. It's what we need to get that feeling-full signal to the brain in a way that carbs just won't do it. That's why more and more people who are successful in achieving and maintaining their ideal weight come to realize and accept the fact that animal protein is a necessity. Animal protein also normalizes blood sugar and gives us a nice smooth energy— not the big burst followed by the all-too-familiar crash that occurs after eating too many carbohydrates.

If we want to live our lives free from addiction, it is imperative that we include animal protein—in many cases, with every meal. Be aware, however, that processed protein such as hot dogs, lunch meats (except some brands of turkey or roast beef), and sausage contain harmful additives as well as large amounts of salt and should definitely be avoided, if possible. Marinate your protein in toasted sesame seed oil and alcohol-free soy sauce mixed with water or a small amount of fresh orange juice and fresh herbs to make it taste delicious.

If you feel very strongly about wanting to eat in a vegetarian way, I understand that being told that you need to eat animal protein can be met with some resistance. Many vegetarians think that they are getting enough protein from soy products or combinations of rice and beans, nuts, or cheese.

However, if you are not getting the results you are seeking, and you have shunned meat for a period of time, I highly recommend that you experiment with adding it into a diet that is already rich with fresh, preferably raw, vegetables and minimal carbohydrate (eaten in a balanced way). Remember, I am not suggesting you eliminate carbohydrate. That rarely works, long term. Simply change the types of carbs you eat to whole-grain and eat them in combination with healthy fat, protein and tons of veggies/salad. Drop the processed, simple carbs and junk from your diet altogether.

Many people are amazed at the results they experience when they make this shift. It's natural to also be concerned about the way the animals are handled, so you may want to look into eating kosher meat or meat that is prepared employing very specific healthful and humane methods. Certainly it's best to select meat that is hormone-free and without antibiotics. Choose high-quality protein sources. Organic, grass-fed beef has 500 percent less saturated fat than feedlot-produced cattle.

There are many people, myself included, who would prefer intellectually, and even taste-wise, to eat in a vegetarian way, Unfortunately, for many of us, our body just doesn't like it. When I don't eat enough animal protein, I simply end up consuming more food. For example, if you gave me the option of a plate filled with yams and brown rice, with a big salad with a delicious tahini (sesame paste) and miso (soy) dressing, as opposed to a rack of lamb with salad, my taste buds would leap in delight at the first option and be totally neutral to the meat.

So we have to be careful with the concept of listening to

our body. What is essential is being aware of which part of our body we are listening to. Sure, my taste buds want the delicious carbs. My mind may even have a brilliant rationale. The first plate is filled with healthy, water-rich food. How can it possibly be bad for me? Plus, consuming grains and vegetables causes no harm to the planet and if I consider the life of the animal, I may even be more inclined to pull back from the idea of a plate of cooked lamb.

However, if I stop and tune in to what my body actually needs, and if I am honest with myself, I will realize that though the dish of complex carbs may be healthful, delicious, nutritious, and satisfying to my taste buds, if I eat them alone without the meat I will probably eat more food than I need to (because the carbs tend to be slow to give the brain the "I'm full—stop eating" signal), and my sweet tooth may very well be triggered to want even more carbs later.

However, if I follow my deeper yearning, it's essential that I look behind the desire for a delicious taste and carbohydrate-filled comfort food. When I instead get in touch with my body's strong, innate need for balance, equilibrium, and health—and I tune in to what satisfies my brain, not just my mouth and emotions—it's clear to me that the type of food that will cut my hunger and curb cravings is animal protein.

I urge you to not feel compelled to either listen to my advice blindly or rebel against it. That just perpetuates the old habit of giving up your power. Instead, I would highly encourage you to experiment, based on the information I'm sharing with you. Even if you have resistance, see what happens in your mind-body when you eat small amounts of animal protein, without chemical-filled sauces, in the way I prescribed. Notice how you feel. Do you feel more satiated? Balanced? Less inclined to want to keep eating? Is it easier to switch gears and get engaged in an activity without going back to wanting more food? It is quite common for people who are prone to sugar addiction, or addiction in general, like you and I, to find that this is the case. For many, eating meat is the number one secret to achieving freedom.

Complex Carbohydrates

Complex carbohydrates are a critical part of our diet. Select from among the following (in combination with protein and healthy fat):

- Whole-grain bread products

- Whole-grain pasta

- Brown rice

- Whole oats

- Barley

- Rye

- Millet

- Whole wheat

Root vegetables such as potatoes, yams, and butternut squash Legumes such as pinto beans, chickpeas, black beans, aduki beans, kidney beans, and soybeans (Although considered to be a source of protein, legumes also are composed of a high level of carbohydrate.)

Carbohydrates aren't "bad"; it's just that if you tend to crave carbohydrates, you need to be really careful with them and eat even the healthy carbs in moderation so they don't start to cause cravings. It's fine to start your day with oatmeal. Don't buy the prepackaged, sugar-filled oatmeal. Instead, it's easy to make from scratch with one part oats to two parts water, with a little bit of sea salt.

To insure a balanced meal and a steadier supply of glucose to your brain, combine the oatmeal with some form of protein such as almond butter or an egg.

Some complex carbohydrates that you can add to your lunch or dinner are whole-grain pasta or brown rice mixed with barley or other grains. You can cook these grains in the organic broths available at your health food store or use the leftover water from your steamed vegetables, which is filled with vitamins and minerals. To cook, add a half cup of any grain to a cup and a half of boiling water or vegetable broth. Allow the dish to simmer until the water is gone.

Other complex carbohydrates are root vegetables such as butternut or acorn squash, potatoes, sweet potatoes, and yams. These are wonderful fiber-, vitamin-, and mineral-rich foods, but make sure to eat them in moderation and combined with greens and animal protein so that you can avoid bingeing. Remember how important it is to be aware of the tendency to substitute one addiction for another. The most likely target for compulsive eating is carbohydrates—even healthy carbohydrates, so use caution.

I recommend that initially you do without bread products as much as possible, but if you really want to have a sandwich, for example, then make sure to use whole-grain or sprouted bread products. Sprouted bread is made from whole-grains or seeds that have been exposed to sun, water, and air. Sprouted grains, beans, and seeds are very high in essential nutrients and are excellent sources of fiber. (A wonderful sandwich idea is sprouted bread with fresh avocado and roasted turkey with fresh green sprouts.)

The more you eat this way, the more you really begin to appreciate the gift of healthier, natural foods. You'll start to realize that the old white flour products, although they taste good, are completely devoid of nutritional value.

Would you fill your car up with water? Of course not, it needs good-quality gasoline and oil to run. Well, your body needs high-nutrition food to be at optimal health. You truly do deserve to eat healthy, water-rich food from the earth. You'll very likely find yourself in deep gratitude for having the opportunity to discover what it feels like to actually honor your body and feed it the life-giving food it craves. The cycle of craving healthy foods begins with switching over and eating those foods and declaring your old way of eating no longer an option for you.

What about Gluten?

Gluten free is the trend right now, but if you've watched nutrition advice over the decades, you've surely noticed that trends with food come and go.

That's why I can't emphasize enough the importance of listening to the wisdom of your own body. I see people go to great lengths to let the world know they are "gluten-free." But I find with all categories of food, what's more important than what you are 'not' eating, is what you 'are' eating. Gluten-free is not synonymous with healthy. There is a lot of gluten free crap out there. Is increasing your corn intake, just because it doesn't have gluten in it, really the wisest course of action?

I highly recommend you tune into what is true for your own body. I don't think everybody should be "gluten-free" necessarily. Yet, there are some people, like those with Celiac Disease, who absolutely must stay away from gluten. My point is this: why eat large amounts of gluten free pizza or gluten free pasta at all? It makes more sense to me, to limit all processed, refined carbs, and eat only complex carbohydrates, in balance with the other categories of food.

If you are going to have something listed in your "moderation" column on your food map, why not enjoy it fully? To me, a treat eaten once in a while is going to taste a lot better if it's made with organic whole wheat rather than some of the alternative flours. Gluten free foods are just as likely to be loaded with sweetener as foods that contain gluten. So unless organic whole wheat is a trigger for you personally, I recommend you select the type of pizza, bread product or homemade "treat" that tastes best to you (with the least amount of sweetener possible), and eat it very sparingly. This way you can fully enjoy it, and are less likely to over-eat.

Ironically, we tend to eat more when we don't fully like what we are eating, and find ourselves seeking "something better or more." When you enjoy some kind of bread/cookie item (preferably one that you bake yourself so you can limit the sweetener to dried fruit, organic apple sauce or coconut) whether it has gluten or not, it's best to eat just the least amount necessary to feel satisfied, and get back to your healthy, balanced, clean eating of veggies, complex carbs, pure protein and omega-3 fat, as soon as possible.

Fats

Another critical component of a healthy diet is fat. Going "low fat" is certainly one of the leading causes of obesity. That's because invariably when you cut out fat, you are going to be eating more sugar. Besides your body requires healthy fat to function optimally. Select the following, preferably organic, in moderation:

- Flaxseed oil

- Extra Virgin Olive oil

- Sesame seed oil

- Avocado

- Coconut Oil

Once you begin choosing healthy fats, you will no longer need to use an abundance of unhealthy sauces. These sauces simply keep the sugar and salt in your system and serve as catalysts to increase your cravings. Be aware, also, of sugar-free substitutes. They often have the exact same effect of stimulating the pancreas and creating the never-ending desire for more sugar. Instead using fresh flaxseed oil or cold-pressed olive oil, with possibly a dash of freshly ground sea salt and/or fresh minced garlic or other herbs such as cilantro, dill, or basil is a wonderful way to flavor your foods.

Some studies suggest that omega-3 fats actually increase your metabolism, improve blood cholesterol levels and turn on messages of weight loss and health in your body. Sources of omega-3 fats are wild salmon, sardines, omega-3 eggs, and extra virgin olive oil and flaxseed oil. In order to retain its nutritional value, flaxseed oil should never be heated.

You can marinate your poultry, meat, and fish in a small amount of high quality, alcohol free soy sauce and toasted sesame seed oil. Don't be afraid to eat healthy fat. Your body needs fat, and when it doesn't get enough of the good fat, it is going to start to crave the bad fat. This dieting mentality is what ultimately leads to bingeing. Even eating some of the fat that comes with the meats you consume can help to ward off binge eating.

Condiments

While condiments are not really a food group, they do add to our enjoyment of food. Select from the following:

- Raw, Organic Apple cider vinegar (with the Mother)

- Sea salt

- Fresh herbs

- Fresh-squeezed lemon

- Slender Cider (see SlenderCider.com)

Foods to Eat in Moderation

If the following are foods you enjoy, and if they are not triggers for you, consume them in moderation. But be cautious, because in general, these are not the healthiest for most people. So why eat them at all?

The challenge with eating only healthy foods like vegetables with protein, is that you could start to feel deprived. So by including some of the foods below, and enough of the healthier carbs, in very moderate amounts, to simply flavor your healthy food and make it taste good, you are increasing the likelihood that you will stick with your sensible eating plan, as a permanent lifestyle.

It's essential that you avoid ever feeling deprived or denied. If you go back to your Food Map, in Chapter Two, you want to make sure that you never feel compelled to eat foods listed on the left of the chart (because they are triggers and precursors to binge eating). Eating foods that you listed in the middle of your Food Map, when you want "something else" is a great way to achieve that. They likely include some of the following:

- Cheese

- Milk

- Canned meats, such as tuna and sardines (high in salt)

- Yogurt

- Canned vegetable juice

- (high in salt) Tofu and other soy products

- Dry-roasted or raw nuts

- Nut butters

- Fruit

- Dried fruit

- Soy milk

- Butter

- Whole-grain flour "healthy" treats

A Balanced Approach: The Craving Cure Modified Eating Plan for Life

When you combine animal protein with salad, vegetables, healthy fat, and a small amount of complex carbohydrate, you have a balanced meal. This is what your body needs. You may need to eat a small, balanced meal every few hours. That's fine. That will keep your blood sugar steady and eliminate any cravings. As far as eating dairy, that's an individual choice and varies case by case. Personally, I eliminated dairy for a long time when I first changed my lifestyle to be free of caffeine, sugar, or alcohol. It took me a while to build my strength back up, and dairy just seemed to aggravate my system.

I still don't like the dairy substitutes, for example soy milk or almond milk, because I find them to be too processed and mostly filled with sweeteners that act as a hunger trigger for me. I really don't miss milk at all and feel much better when it's out of my system. Over time, I have been able to reincorporate some cheese back into my diet, which I enjoy regularly. Remember, the key to ultimate success is enjoying the foods that you eat, and sometimes dairy or nuts, in moderation, give the food just the zest it needs to help you avoid craving the foods that are much more harmful to you.

Keep track of the effect foods such as dairy have on you with a food inventory. Log the foods you are eating and how you feel before you eat them and after. This will help to give you a sense of which foods agree with you and which foods are best avoided. Perhaps you will be able to eat certain foods that used to trigger cravings, in moderation, in the future. Only you will be able to determine that. Experiment with how you feel both when you eat the questionable food and when you don't. Some people notice a difference in their overall mood and energy level when they eat cheese, for example, and some don't. It's the same thing with fruit. Some people do fine with one or two pieces of fruit a day, and others notice an intense increase in sugar cravings and hunger in general when fruit is in their system. So take the time to learn about your unique body and how it responds to various foods.

Avoiding Common Mistakes

A common pitfall when giving up a vice is to substitute an equally harmful habit. Unfortunately, all you are doing with that tactic is delaying the inevitable cleansing that your body needs to do in order to repair itself and be fully restored to health and vitality. The first addiction I let go of was alcohol. The day I stopped drinking alcohol was the day I started drinking massive amounts of caffeine.

When I finally began to see that sugar was a major problem for me, I did stop eating it, however, I replaced it with sugar substitutes— completely oblivious to the greater health risks associated with these chemical substances. I also started to take diet pills. It wasn't until I lost all my energy and could barely get out of bed in the morning that I got serious and admitted to myself that I had been simply substituting one harmful addiction for another. I realized that I was going to have to not only make minor alterations in my diet, but instead, radically shift the way I thought about food (and substances).

When I cut out all the unhealthy stimulants and simplified my diet by selecting whole, unprocessed foods, lots of vegetables, whole-grain products, healthy fats, and small amounts of anti-biotic and hormone free animal protein, my health entirely turned around. I could see that what used to seem like normal food to me before was to a great extent toxic and bogging down my whole system. Of course, it's not always going to be possible to eat whole, unprocessed foods. I do find, though, that a commitment to taking care of myself and making health my priority helps me to make the best choices available in any given situation, while at the same time being able to live in a world where processed food is often the norm. We don't want to eliminate categories of food, because that can also set us up for cravings—but rather choose healthier versions.

Tune In to the Benefit of Living Sugar-Free

Now, before you despair and start entertaining any ideas about how boring it is to eat this way, realize that this is just a picture in your mind. In reality, healthful foods can be absolutely satisfying and taste delicious. You may also be concerned about the time involved in preparing such foods. I want to assure you that once you change your habits, the time it takes to put them together is minimal. Some of your apprehension is simply a natural fear of change and a certain comfort level with eating the way you do.

It's likely that the majority of the foods you crave fall into the simple carbohydrate category. It simply boils down to the fact that the foods we are most likely to be addicted to are simple carbohydrates, containing sugar, white flour, and/or caffeine. Even an addiction to alcohol is in a way an addiction to sugar. Many alcoholics stop drinking booze only to substitute large quantities of sugar or cigarettes.

If you stopped smoking you may notice that you began to substitute sweet foods. This is because even cigarettes are laced with addictive additives and sweet flavors. It's important to open your awareness of these things so that you can outsmart your addictions. Otherwise you will feebly go from one addiction to the next. You may let go of your after-dinner dish of ice cream, only to replace this habit with a bowl of potato chips or popcorn or a Diet Coke. Look at what your body is craving—it's that sweet taste. Even though the Diet Coke has no calories, it stimulates your body to want more sweet or stimulating food. Caffeine works on the same principle. The more of the stimulating, sweet foods you eat, the stronger your craving for more of the same.

Foods to Eliminate

- Sugar (including fructose, maltose, dextrose, maple syrup, molasses, glucose, honey)

- High-fructose corn syrup

- Sugar substitutes

- Mayonnaise

- Catsup

- White bread

- White flour bagels

- White rice

- White flour pasta

- Commercial cookies or candy

- Ice cream

- Cake

- Soda or soft drinks

- Chocolate

- Cream

- Frozen yogurt

- Caffeine

- Diet pills

- Vegetable oils (processed and hydrogenated)

- Margarine

- Table salt

- Processed fruit juice (high in sugar, albeit fructose)

- Spreads

- Salad dressing

- (store-bought) Barbecue sauce

- Relish

- Salted nuts roasted in oil

- Frankfurters

- Sausage

- Cold cuts

- Alcohol

When you look at the list of foods to avoid, it may feel over-whelming, as this list is likely to include many items that you are used to eating every day. I want to assure you that after you go on the Two-Week Mega-Nutrition Cleanse (described in Chapter 11) and get these foods out of your system, they will simply not have the same appeal for you. The cleanse will remove much of your desire to eat foods that lack nutritional value, trigger hunger, or create disease in your system.

Transitioning to Healthier Foods

If you go to your health food store and read the labels, you can find healthier, more natural versions of catsup, mayonnaise, and salad dressing. If you feel that getting rid of everything at once will cause you to feel panicked that there's nothing to eat, you can substitute these healthier versions, as a stepping-stone, in the interim. However, I recommend that you ultimately cut back on these fattening, empty-calorie condiments in general, because even the healthier versions are very likely to cause your food cravings to persist. After your cleanse, it will be easier to determine which foods are safe for you to reintroduce into your diet, without leading you back to food addiction.

Eating in a simpler way, selecting whole foods in their natural state as much as possible, is what is going to free you from the endless cycle of compulsive eating. Adding small amounts of sesame oil with some sea salt can give your food just the right amount of flavor so that you enjoy it fully, without being set up for insatiable hunger. Also, as I mentioned earlier, it's OK to use dry-roasted nuts and perhaps a small amount of cheese to flavor your food. Again, these foods must be used in moderation. For some people, the foods listed in the "Foods to Eat in Moderation" list are fine, but for others, they need to be avoided completely because they lead to cravings or overeating.

Don't worry if you are unsure about which items may have a negative effect on you. After you complete your Two-Week Mega-Nutrition Cleanse (see Chapter 11), it will be easier for you to determine if you can get away with the foods in this category or whether they cause you to binge. Certainly, if you are going to choose to eat these foods, read the labels and select the brands with the least amount of sweeteners, sodium, and additives.

In summary, if you suffer from incessant food cravings, the foods to eat regularly are mostly dark greens and other vegetables, mixed with animal protein, healthy fats, and smaller amounts of complex carbohydrates. Also remember to do the following:

- **Eat in a balanced way.** Find and eat foods that you like. It's essential that you enjoy the foods you eat; otherwise, you are bound to keep searching for something else to satisfy you. Balance your intake of protein, fresh vegetables, healthy fat, and carbohydrate.

- **Avoid excessive fruit.** Fruit, if tolerated, can be eaten in moderation.

- **Drink water.** Lots of fresh, pure water is important because it will cleanse your system, fill you up and help to free you from any kind of food or substance addiction. Often thirst is misinterpreted as hunger. Most people do not drink enough water. It's recommended that you drink half your body weight in ounces. So if you weigh 200 pounds, it would be best if you drank 100 ounces of filtered water daily. Reach for water throughout the day.

- **Remember to exercise.** Physical activity is essential to increase your metabolic rate and improve your sense of well-being. See Chapter 6 for creative ideas on increasing daily movement and making it fun.

- **Eat breakfast daily.** Studies show that people who skip breakfast are much more likely to overeat later in the day.

- **Eat regularly.** Your body needs to trust that when it gets hungry, you will care for it and feed it. It's often the unconscious fear that you won't get your true needs met that causes overeating and bingeing when you are not physically hungry. Regular meals throughout the day help you to maintain a steady blood sugar level. Feed your body when it's physically hungry the way a mother would tend to her new baby.

- **Snack smartly.** If you're hungry between meals, munch on raw carrots and celery, with some animal protein such as a hard-boiled egg or a thin slice of roast beef.

- **Marinate.** Instead of buying processed lunch meat, roast your own turkey. Rather than cover it in prepared barbecue sauce filled with sodium and sugar, marinate the fresh turkey in sesame seed oil and high quality, alcohol free soy sauce.

- **Satisfy your sweet tooth.** If you have a strong desire for a sweet taste, experiment with adding a few raisins and chopped dry-roasted nuts to your vegetables or whole-grains.

- **Experiment with salads.** If you prefer to change your eating habits gradually, simply begin by adding a huge green salad to go along with the meals you typically eat. Make the salad, lightly dressed with extra virgin olive oil dressing, the main focus of the meal, adding your regular dish on the side or on top of the salad for flavor instead of focusing on your main dish and perhaps just having a small salad on the side.

(Checkout my 4 minute video demonstration on how
to easily make the healthiest, delicious salad dressing,
on my Blog at EasyWillpower.com).

Years of abuse in terms of addictive behaviors around food,
diet pills, drugs or alcohol have very likely skewed your natural signals of what is right or wrong for you. Therefore, be
patient and give your body some time to readjust and normalize. The cleaner you can keep your system on the inside,
the easier it will be for your body to heal and purify itself.
In the next three chapters, you will learn methods that will
help you immensely to speed up this cleansing process. The
Two-Week Mega-Nutrition Cleanse, coming up in Chapter
11, will also assist you in discovering and eliminating any
food sensitivities that are triggering hunger and perpetuating cravings.

But first, I want to share with you some exciting news
about a nutrient we are hearing more and more about: CBD.
CBD is most known for its ability to help alleviate pain,
improve sleep, and as a treatment for Epilepsy, along with a
host of other ailments. It's true that high quality, pharmaceutical grade CBD can be used medicinally to treat many
conditions, including Diabetes. What I am most excited about
is how CBD can assist people in breaking free from addiction. Another promising discovery I've made is how it can
be paired with other ingredients to help achieve healthy
weight loss and fewer cravings for harmful substances. In
Chapter Nine, you'll discover how to incorporate a powerful Cannabinoid herb into your diet—CBD—to help you find
mind-body balance and eliminate cravings and addiction.

9. The Truth About CBD

It's almost impossible to live on this planet and not have heard about CBD in recent months. What is CBD? Is it a fad? A miracle drug? Does it have any value at all? These are great questions. Other valid concerns are, if I want to try CBD, how do I know who and what brand to trust? How much should I take? Why do I need it? What forms do CBD come in and what's the best way to take it? How does it even work? Will it interact with my medications? Or, I tried CBD, why didn't it work for me?

These are excellent questions that I am happy to answer for you. First, let me start by telling you what CBD is and how I came to discover it, myself.

CBD stands for Cannabidiol. Cannabidiol comes from the same plant that Marijuana is derived from—the Cannabis plant. You could say that CBD and Marijuana are cousins—but there is a huge, important difference. CBD does not make you high. Marijuana contains THC which has a psychoactive component. By contrast, CBD does not make you high, yet it is shown to have strong medicinal compounds. In fact, over 20,000 medical and clinical studies have been conducted on CBD and published in scientific journals. Not only does CBD not get you high, it's been reported to be an effective antidote to THC because it actually reduces the psychoactive effects of THC. Nowadays, there is a vast, consistent movement across the United States and throughout the world to legalize marijuana, particularly medical marijuana. But it's important to understand that this is a separate issue because CBD is not marijuana and it does not get you high.

States that have legalized medical marijuana require that you have a medical prescription or license to purchase medical marijuana. Though CBD comes from the same plant family, CBD, legally known as Industrial Hemp, requires no medical license. In other words, anyone, in any of the 50 states can take CBD, 100% legally. CBD can be shipped across state lines, legally. This all began in 2014 when President Obama signed the Farm Bill. Prior to that, CBD had been considered illegal for political reasons, for decades. In December 2018, both political parties in the United States Government, as well as the President, passed the newest Farm Bill, once again confirming that CBD is completely legal.

Why CBD?

As a health and wellness expert and corporate speaker presenting weight loss and smoking cessation seminars in hospitals for decades, I had been approached many times by supplement companies. Nutriceutical executives often reached out to me, requesting that I endorse their brand. Even though I am a big advocate of natural herbs and the medicinal power of plants, I had no interest in promoting supplements. In fact, for the first 20 years of presenting in hospital settings, I never sold any dietary supplements at all. I was always a firm believer in getting your required nutrients from food. I also happen to be super sensitive to most substances and can't take them, even if they do have value. So there hadn't been anything I felt comfortable endorsing. My message was strictly teaching people how to tap into the vast power of the subconscious mind, through a form of self-hypnosis, to change their habits and create massive life changing results.

Then, about 10 years back, I noticed some changes in my own body as I entered the next decade of life. I had gained about 5 pounds even though I had not deviated from my healthful eating and exercise plan that I had adopted since getting healthy in my late twenties. I didn't want to go on any kind of diet, and I was very cautious about increasing activity, with my history of over-exercising, when I had been younger.

I started experimenting with herbs for energy, metabolism and digestion, along with organic apple cider vinegar. To my surprise, Slender Cider, was born. My clients, friends and family absolutely loved my new creation and encouraged me to bring it to market. It took me a year of pounding the pavement throughout the country, to find an organic manufacturer, with a level of integrity I was truly comfortable with. I wanted to be sure that all the herbs were fresh brewed just like a cup of tea, without powders and fillers to cheapen the product. I've been so delighted with the Slender Cider I was able to bring to market. It has helped so many of my clients to lose weight, in addition to my hypnotherapy systems, because it helps alkalize, cleanse and energize on a physical level. Slender Cider is a liquid, herbal concentrate of 11 therapeutic herbs in a base of organic apple cider vinegar. You just mix it with water and sip it throughout the day. My customers love the way it tastes—clean, healthy and natural.

Up until this past year, Slender Cider was the only supplement I felt comfortable recommending to my following, because it's so gentle to the system and it contains only premium and organic ingredients.

New Information

All that changed in the summer of 2016 when my doctor informed me that my Glaucoma was getting worse. I had been diagnosed about 8 years prior, and was very concerned because since I had contracted the disease, I had already lost a lot of vision that could never be recovered. Glaucoma is an illness where the pressures in the eyes are remarkably high, causing death to the optic nerve, resulting in permanent loss of vision. When the ophthalmologist informed me that I would need surgery and increased medication, he got my attention. Even though western medicine had saved my life with a pacemaker at the age of 26, I was not in a hurry to start taking pharmaceutical drugs nor did I want to have any surgery.

About that time, my husband, who is an acupuncture physician with a keen interest in the benefits of medical marijuana, said to me, "Why don't you try CBD?" Over the years, he had encouraged me to experiment with Cannabis to decrease my eye pressures (marijuana is known to help Glaucoma), but I had always refused. I did not want to put anything psychoactive in my body. With my history of addiction to various substances, I was determined to stay clear of any possibly mind altering elements.

In that moment, my options seemed limited. It was evident that I needed to stabilize the pressures in my eyes, or risk losing even more vision. Skeptical, I decided to try CBD, since there was no psychoactive component to it. I was so pleasantly surprised by what I discovered. I started sleeping more soundly. My hormones felt much more balanced. I experienced deeper relaxation throughout the day and best of all, my doctor informed me that my eye pressures were lower than ever. I no longer needed surgery or increased medication for my eyes.

I wanted to shout out about this miracle substance from the rooftops. I set out to investigate the best source of CBD products so I could inform my clients. What I discovered shocked me. The world of CBD was like the wild, wild West.

Sure there were many people touting the benefits, from

Internet sales people to local doctors in my community. But the marketing information being shared was very deceiving.

Quality is Everything

In the meantime, I worked very hard to source high quality CBD, so I could share it with my own following. Though I had not set out to create my own line of CBD products, that's exactly what ended up happening.

As I shared my high quality CBD with my clients who were not only wanting to lose weight, but were also begging for relief from physical pain, anxiety, insomnia, and in many cases, addiction; the stories they relayed to me were so gratifying. At the same time, I came to see more and more how important it is for people to be informed before spending their hard-earned money on CBD.

For example, I had one client who ended up buying my Rena's Organic 1000 mg. CBD Pain Relief Cream bringing me the CBD Salve he had previously purchased from his neurologist. I looked at the bottle and no-where on the label did it report how many milligrams of CBD were in the bottle. I called the physician's office and was told that "no-one reveals how much CBD is in their product." I assured the receptionist that this was not the case and that patients needed to be informed as to how much CBD they are taking. Clearly, the amount of CBD in the doctor's lotion was so miniscule, it was more convenient to leave the amount off the label. Even so, my client had paid the doctor over $100 for that useless "CBD" cream.

Chiropractors throughout the country are selling a brand of CBD with impressive, medical-looking packaging. The jars are labeled Level One through Level Five. Again, no-where on the packaging is the potency of CBD revealed. After careful analysis of the CBD brand's website, we saw that Level One contained a ridiculous 25 mg. of CBD and their Level Five, which sold for $80, had only 200 mg. of CBD. That's when I knew I had to speak out to protect vulnerable people from getting ripped off.

It took me over a year to bring my products to market, but it finally happened a few months back. It's such a thrill to get comments from my customers, telling me that the pain they had lived with for years, is "just gone," as so many report. That's because my CBD pain relief creams have 500 mg. CBD and 1000 mg. CBD. There's just no point in using weaker potencies if you want to experience true relief. And the best part is, due to cost-saving measures and keeping the overhead low at my company, I'm able to sell my 500 mg. CBD Pain Relief Cream for the same price or less than Chiropractors are selling their 200 mg. CBD pain cream for! And I make sure that the Rena's Organic pain relief and beauty creams (CBD is amazing for the skin) are using full spectrum CBD rather than cheap isolate. Keep reading to learn more about that.

How Does CBD Work?

In the late 1980's, a group of scientists discovered the Endo-cannabinoid System in the human body. The Endocannabinoid System (ECS) is a connected system of ligands, receptors and enzymes and is present throughout your entire body. In fact, all mammals have an endocannabinoid system. According to scientists, the endo-cannabinoid system is essential to your survival, and your body can't function without it. That's because it regulates every significant biological function in the body. In a nutshell, your endo-cannabinoid system controls how you eat, sleep, relax and even helps your memory. It also regulates metabolism and mood.

Many health problems, including all addiction and food addiction in particular, are caused by or exacerbated by the body's inability to achieve homeostasis or balance. When your ECS is not functioning optimally, you will experience an imbalance. That could lead to digestive disorders, fatigue, brain fog, hormones out of whack, depression, anxiety, and a host of other ailments, including weight gain and cravings.

The body doesn't see cannabinoids as a foreign substance or drug. Rather it recognizes cannabinoids as natural signaling molecules that are essential for optimal health. There are two types of cannabinoids. Endo-cannabinoids are our endogenous cannabinoids—those that the body produces naturally. Phyto-cannabinoids, on the other hand, are plant cannabinoids. The body recognizes plant-derived cannabinoids as valuable compounds that are essential for various functions. The body doesn't "crave" cannabinoids, or become addicted to them. It simply needs cannabinoids in the same way that it requires a full range of minerals and vitamins. There are many plant cannabinoids, but the strongest and most effective plant cannabinoid is CBD from the Industrial Hemp or Cannabis plant. CBD actually mimics the action of naturally occurring endo-cannabinoids in the human body.

Endo-cannibinoid receptor cells are found throughout the body, which is why so many bodily systems are effected by the cannabinoids within. Research is showing that our bodies need cannabinoids to achieve homeostasis. Since your body naturally produces it's own Endo-cannabinoids, why do we need to ingest cannabinoids?

Cannabinoid deficiency is a fairly recent phenomenon and is most likely so prevalent because of the heavily processed diet most people are consuming. Science is also pointing to the modern stressful lifestyle and lack of exercise as factors that could be contributing to the syndrome known as clinical cannabinoid deficiency. It's evident that previously unknown illnesses are affecting society much more prevalently than in the past. Take cancer for example. On the block I grew up on in Somerset, New Jersey, there was only one person that we knew of who had contracted cancer. I remember what a shock it was. Fast forward a few decades. It's unlikely that you or I know any family that has NOT been impacted by cancer! While there are a multitude of factors that may be contributing to the prevalence of an increase in many illnesses and diseases, it makes sense that a deficiency in the endo-cannabinoid system could be contributing. CBD helps to replenish the ECS receptors.

Though the body produces its own Cannabinoids, an enzyme known as the FAAH (fatty acid amide hydrolase) enzyme decreases the life span of the endo-cannabinoids, throughout the body. It acts as a little "pac-man" metabolizing cannabinoids, thereby limiting their availability. Therefore, adding plant cannabinoids to your diet, increases the amount of cannabinoids available to attach to the receptor cells throughout the body.

According to researchers, CBD has the ability to link up with receptor cells in every system of the body. The main function of the Endo-cannabinoid system is to bring homeostasis or balance to the body. A stressful lifestyle and a diet void of high nutrition has likely created an imbalance in your body's systems. The function of the Endo-cannabinoid system is to bring balance back to the whole body, including your nervous system, digestive system, cardiovascular system and endocrine system. CBD has been shown to mimic some of the modulating endo-cannabinoid system receptors that regulate neuro-transmitters or an overactive immune response. CBD has been shown to connect with receptors at the mitochondria and nucleus to increase energy production while protecting the cell from reactive oxygen damage. That's why CBD can produce amazing healing results for such a wide variety of health conditions—both mental, emotional and physical—because it is creating a positive shift at the cellular level, thus increasing cellular energy.

The cannabinoids in CBD activate key CB1 and CB2 receptors. These receptors work to regulate hormonal activity which is why CBD can help reduce pain and anxiety while improving sleep and libido. The CB2 receptor is found primarily in the immune system. An immune system that is not functioning properly is going to impact every other system in the body including the cardiovascular system, digestive system, endocrine system, the central nervous system as well as all the tissues and organs in your body.

You may wonder, how can CBD be reported to help so many ailments? The answer is because the endo-cannabinoid system is not limited to any one, specific area of bodily function. When I started to ingest CBD to help manage my Glaucoma, I never expected the other side "benefits".

The research on CBD has shown that taking CBD orally and using high-potency CBD creams topically can offer dramatic relief from painful spasms and muscle stiffness. It's truly gratifying to see people who were once in pain able to perform their daily activities pain-free and enjoy a much higher quality of life. Pharmaceutical grade, full spectrum CBD is being used very effectively for arthritic pain all over the body because it has the ability to link up with receptors that control pain and inflammation. In fact, one of the most known attributes of CBD is its ability to reduce inflammation. That's why CBD is so valuable for pain control as well as for treating ailments like diabetes. Not only does CBD assist in the treatment of diabetes due to it's inflammatory reducing properties, but also because endo-cannabinoids have the ability to regulate insulin release.

For this reason, CBD is also very beneficial in balancing blood sugar and improving digestion and elimination, as well as reducing brain fog.

Further evidence on the potential efficacy of CBD is the fact that the United States Government has taken out a patent on it. The patent acknowledges CBD as a powerful anti-seizure, anti-oxidant and anti-inflammatory, pointing to remarkable benefits that protect your entire body, from cellular damage from free radicals. A free radical is an oxygen molecule that has split off into unpaired electrons. Since electrons want to be paired in order to feel stable, these "loose" electrons scavenge the body, seeking to pair up. In the process they cause what's known as "oxidative stress," causing serious damage to DNA and the body's cells.

Why the Controversy?

If CBD can even offer half of the benefits it's being reported to help, why on earth is there any controversy around it at all?

As early as 2700 BC, ancient civilizations, including the Greeks, used this natural healing compound to treat pain, anxiety, inflammation, insomnia, memory loss, skin diseases and a host of other ailments. The Chinese were using it as medicine thousands of years ago. From the 1850s all the way through 1900, CBD was used by physicians throughout the United States as a trusted remedy for over 100 distinct diseases. Even George Washington, our founding Father, grew hemp at his home in Virginia.

CBD has been reported to be safe, amazingly effective and

non-addictive. Doctors and scientists have known about the healing properties in this plant compound for decades. But the United States Government put an end to its use in the early part of last century. That's because in 1937, this healing herb was caught up in legislation that made it illegal to grow, buy or use. You may wonder, if CBD is made from Hemp, and it doesn't make you "high", why was it banned all these years? The story is this: In 1937, congress passed a law that made it illegal to grow Cannabis in the United States. Because Hemp is part of the same plant family, it became illegal to grow Hemp as well. Thankfully, due to new regulations, this ban has been lifted.

Nowadays, doctors are paying attention to their patients and recommending CBD, to some extent. My ophthalmologist never asked me what I did to control my eye pressures and had no interest in discussing CBD. On the other hand, now that I've created my own brand of CBD products at RenasOrganic.com, I am so impressed with the number of physicians who send their patients to me for their CBD products. I've had more than one doctor, including neurologists, acupuncturists and chiropractors, confess that it's still very challenging for them to know where to get high quality CBD.

One neurologist in our community, who treats a lot of Parkinson's Disease, was sending her patients to a local pharmacy to get CBD pills. However, she reported back to us that her patients who were taking the Rena's Organic 1500 mg. CBD tincture were actually improving at a higher rate, and the physician discontinued sending her patients to the pharmacy.

The British Journal of Clinical Pharmacology reported that "CBD can relieve the tingling, burning and discomfort of neuropathy—and does it without effecting memory or nerve function." Because so many of my clients suffer from depression, what fascinated me most about CBD was its mood enhancing benefits. I was particularly intrigued that the United States Military was using it successfully for PTSD—an ailment that one in five military personnel suffers from. According to a study reported by the National Institute of health, people who suffer from anxiety or PTSD have low levels of certain receptors in their Endo-cannabinoid system—especially the receptors that control stress, fear and memories. CBD has been known to replenish these missing receptors and bring the endo-cannabinoid system and the whole body back into homeostasis—or healthy balance.

Why is it so challenging to find high quality CBD?

The great news is that CBD is now accessible to all of us. The bad news is that the industry is completely unregulated. CBD products are springing up everywhere. CBD tinctures are even available at my local gas station!

CBD comes in many forms: pills, capsules, vapes and oils. You'll also find CBD infused gummies, chocolates and candy. Recently a few States including New York outlawed adding CBD to coffee and food, in convenience stores and coffee shops. CBD is available as a dietary or herbal supplement, across state lines. If you want to order CBD online and use CBD medicinally for optimal health, mentally, physically and emotionally, it's essential that you become a smart shopper.

How can you know what CBD is best for you?

Let's look at bio-availability, purity of product, how it was grown and extracted, and other ingredients, if any, that comprise various CBD products.

First of all, it's helpful to realize that real CBD is an expensive ingredient. It's costly to grow and extract high quality CBD. When CBD products are priced very low, you may wonder, how is this possible?

There are 7 things to look for when buying CBD:

1. What is the potency?

2. Is it Full Spectrum?

3. Is it true Cannabidiol (CBD) or is it just Hemp?

4. Is it USA, organically grown, from seed to shelf?

5. How is it extracted?

6. What other ingredients, if any, are paired with the CBD?

7. Does the brand you selected have a 3rd party test analysis that you can view?

Let's look at each of these factors. But first let's address a very common question: How much CBD should I take?

Determining How Much CBD to Take

The reality is, there is no one dosage that is perfect for everyone. When starting out with CBD, it's best to begin by taking just a few milligrams at a time. So for example, if you were to take a 300 mg. tincture, a full dropper would be 10 mg. That may be a perfect dose for you to start. Ideally, you would divide the dose, so that you are taking your CBD a few times a day. For example, you may start out with a few drops in the morning, a couple drops in the afternoon and a 3-4 more drops at bedtime. The advantage of a tincture is that you can take it sublingually, meaning under the tongue. This accelerates the speed at which the CBD enters your bloodstream, because you are bypassing the digestive process.

Many people, especially when using CBD medicinally, need to take a higher potency to get the results they are looking for. But over time, it's not uncommon to actually reduce your dosage and still maintain the medicinal effects you are seeking. People using CBD to help combat inflammation or arthritic pain, often do better with higher potencies. When I was in acute pain, twice, from pulling my back out, I reached for the Rena's Organic 1500 mg. CBD Tincture, with amazing results. I actually took 3-4 full droppers throughout the day. A full dropper of 1500 mg. CBD tincture has 50 mg. CBD. That may seem like a lot, especially when it's such high quality, full spectrum CBD. When an individual is in pain, the body can tolerate a much higher dose than would otherwise be necessary. At the same time, I applied the 1000 mg. CBD Pain Relief Cream to my lower back, with amazing results. When the acute pain subsided, in a day or two, I could reduce my dose drastically and still maintain the benefits. It's been so gratifying to hear from so many people who are having similar pain relief experiences using either the 1000 mg CBD pain relief cream on its own, or combined with the Full Spectrum oils.

I recommend, when you are first beginning to take CBD orally, that you take it in the evening before bed. One of the greatest benefits of CBD is that it helps you to fall asleep. It's an incredible aid for insomnia, whether you have trouble falling asleep or staying asleep. Though there are no known risks to taking CBD, and it is considered to be completely safe, a potential "side-effect" for some could be fatigue. That's why medical grade CBD is such a great option to help you to fall asleep at night. But it's for this reason that I recommend that you start out taking CBD in the evening, just in case you get sleepy. As your body gets used to CBD, your needs may change, and you may find that you do well taking CBD throughout the day. In fact, most people who enjoy the benefits of CBD do take it throughout the day as it really helps to reduce the effects of stress and "take the edge off."

It's best to start out with a conservative dose and build up from there when taking CBD orally. When applying CBD topically, such as when using CBD pain relief cream, it's fine to apply liberally. However, when you are using a high quality, high potency CBD lotion or salve, it's likely that only a small amount will give you the results that you are seeking. People are using CBD topically for relief from neuropathy, muscle spasms and all kinds of acute and chronic pain.

Potency

Even though it's a good idea to start out with small amounts of CBD so that your body can get used to it, when shopping for CBD, it's very important that you read your label to fully understand potency. Sadly, there is a lot of deception when it comes to CBD labeling, even when the CBD is being sold in reputable places (like doctor's offices!). Intentional or not, the reality is that CBD label confusion and misinformation, is the norm. As a customer, it's up to you to do your research.

What's the Difference Between CBD and Hemp

For example, a bottle may be labeled as 1000 mg. Hemp. Hemp and CBD may be terms that are used interchangeably, but there is a huge difference between the two compounds. You can not assume that if a bottle is labeled 1000 mg. Hemp, there are 1000 mg. of CBD or Cannabidiol in that bottle. It can be very confusing because all CBD is also known as Industrial Hemp. However, all Hemp is NOT CBD. Hemp could just be Hemp Seed. Though Hemp Seed Oil has value, just like Olive Oil and Grape Seed Oil, Hemp Seed Oil is not medicinal in nature. Albeit Hemp Seed Oil is a healthy oil, it is the CBD itself that carries the medicinal qualities of the plant, not Hemp Seed Oil. When purchasing CBD, you want to make sure that the bottle label states that you are getting at least 250 mg. CBD in the bottle, and if you are treating a medical condition, you most likely would like to get an even stronger potency than that.

Why Full Spectrum Makes a Difference

Full spectrum means that the product is derived from the whole plant, as opposed to just an isolated component of the plant. It's essential to only use CBD products that are organically grown and that utilize the entire plant. That's because the different parts of the plant work synergistically with each other to create the medicinal benefits. Full Spectrum products mean that the CBD has all the cannabinoids, chlorophyll, flavenoids and terpenes in the plant. A terpene is a plant essential oil that retains medicinal attributes.

In 2018, the World Health Organization stated clearly that "naturally occurring" CBD is safe and well-tolerated in people and animals with no negative effects. Full Spectrum CBD is naturally occurring. What I've seen with some product labeling is a very high potency – for example, 1000 mg. or 1500 mg. CBD tincture, but upon close examination, it's evident that even if some full spectrum CBD is in the product, it is then spiked with much cheaper, CBD isolate, to bring up the potency number.

As the name implies, CBD isolate is typically isolated with a chemical, solvent based method. Isolates are made with a harsh extraction process that strip vital phyto-nutrients from the plant. The difference between CBD isolates and whole plant, lipid infused CBD is huge. For the highest level of medical efficacy, you'll want to stick with Full Spectrum CBD. A word of caution: By definition, legally, full spectrum CBD contains less than .3% THC. THC stands for tetrahydrocannabinol and is the component of the marijuana plant that is responsible for its psychoactive effects. At the strength of less than point three percent, the purpose of the THC in full spectrum CBD is simply to help activate the healing potential of the entire plant. Remember it's the synergy of taking the entire plant—flower, leaves, stem, seeds—all of it, that yields the miraculous healing effects that is making CBD the new buzz word in health. In those tiny amounts (less than .3%), the THC helps to bring out the medicinal value of the CBD and other Cannabinoids but will not make you high.

Where is Your CBD Grown?

The Cannabis plant, from which CBD is derived, is a very porous plant. That means that it has the potential to absorb toxins from the earth and from the environment where it's grown. That's why it's essential that you only buy CBD that is grown in a regulated State.

Many CBD sellers cut expenses by buying and selling CBD that is sourced overseas. Even if the CBD is then processed in the United States, the seeds themselves may have come from China. CBD products grown in Europe frequently originate from seeds that have been sent over from Asia. Why is this a problem? Because there are few regulatory conditions on the toxicity of the water, soil and air in that part of the world.

It's essential that your CBD be clean and pure and organically grown. I will only use CBD that is organically grown, from seed to shelf, in Colorado. It is very comforting to know that the regulations for growing Cannabis in Colorado are very high. The weather conditions are also perfect. I also only would source from a farm that is growing according to organic specifications, with certifications to back that up. In fact, it took me months to find a reputable CBD farm that I could trust completely to not only meet but exceed the potencies necessary for medical grade CBD.

Additionally, when a farm uses its own proprietary

genetic strands of Cannabis, the products are consistent from batch to batch. By far, CBD, organically grown from a reputable farm in Colorado, is not the least expensive CBD at all, but when it comes to health it makes absolutely no sense to cut corners. Top quality, high potency CBD is worth every penny. And if you can cut back on your medications, with your doctor's permission of course, as you get healthier, it will certainly be worth your higher quality of life (and the money you save on pharmaceuticals)!

Extraction

The most expensive and the cleanest, most efficient extraction method is Super Critical CO2 Extraction. Ethanol extraction is less expensive but often leaves heavy chemical residues on the plant. Super Critical CO2 is an extraction process that is food-approved, natural and non-toxic. Because it is a clean extraction process, it protects the plant material during extraction. Beware of chemical residues in your CBD product, depending on how it was extracted. The label should reveal that information.

What Ingredients are Paired with Your CBD?

An important consideration when taking CBD for your health is, what other ingredients are mixed in with the CBD? Gummies and CBD infused candy of one kind or another have become the rage.

While CBD has been proven to be safe and non-toxic, I would be equally concerned about the chemicals and flavorings that may be mixed in. Same with vaping. Vaping is becoming increasingly popular. Aside from the studies revealing the health risks of vaping to the lungs, and other bodily systems, for those of us committed to leading an addiction-free life, my bigger concern is the flavorings and chemicals that are inherent in all vape products. It's for this reason that my brand, Rena's Organic, does not carry any vaping products.

I am committed to only sharing products that have been found to increase health on every level. So even though vape advocates report that vaping is the fastest way to get CBD into the bloodstream, there are too many risks there for people with a history of any kind of addiction. That's because the chemicals and additives in vape oil are no better than the chemicals in cigarettes. A wonderful alternative is high potency CBD oil, in tinctures, that you drop under the tongue and that are comprised of nothing more than omega-3 MCT (fractionated coconut) oil, and possibly a drop of organic essential oil.

Breaking Free from Addiction

My greatest commitment is to helping people who have been struggling with addiction. To me, the number one barrier to health and happiness is addiction of one form or another. That's why, when I discovered CBD, I wanted to pair it with only the healthiest ingredients, to increase mental, physical and emotional health. I have been really excited to bring to market two amazing products that do just that.

CBD Super Cider is an amazing health tonic that helps alkalize and cleanse while increasing the benefits of CBD. Though it wasn't easy to get the organic certification, CBD Super Cider is one of the only USDA certified organic CBD products on the market.

It contains 400 mg. full spectrum CBD in Hemp Seed Oil, in a base of organic apple cider vinegar and organic cherry concentrate. It is blended with a very powerful herbal formula, of 7 Cannabinoid herbs. These herbs work synergistically, to increase the efficacy of CBD. Remember I told you that there are other Phyto-Cannabinoid herbs, but CBD is the strongest one? Other herbs that benefit your Endo-Cannabinoid system, that are in CBD Super Cider, are Turmeric, Echinacea, Helichrysum, Black Pepper, Nutmeg, Cinnamon and Cacao. Each of these herbs is known to contain phyto-cannabinoid properties. You can certainly increase your consumption of those herbs independently, by adding them to your diet. Each one is a powerhouse of nutrition and also works to balance your endo-cannabinoid system.

When you plan your high nutrition cleanse that you'll be learning about in an upcoming chapter, it's a great idea to incorporate these healthy, balancing cannabinoid herbs.

Another wonderful way I have found to pair medical grade CBD is with super foods, super greens and herbs. CBD Super Food contains 250 mg. water soluble CBD, which gives it increased bio-availability, blended with 23 other organic super foods, including greens, herbs and berries. My clients love this powder because it's so easy to mix into a glass of water. It tastes great but it's not too sweet. One of the problems with so many supplements on the market, especially powders, drinks and smoothies is that they are sickeningly sweet. I literally sent my formula back to my co-packer 9 times because I was committed to toning down the sweetness. I feel strongly about this, even though I understand that Stevia is a healthy sweetener. Studies show that high quality Stevia actually balances blood sugar. Nevertheless, in my own experience and working with so many thousands of people struggling with addiction, I have found that it's the sweet taste itself that prolongs sugar cravings and addiction. Even the sweet taste of healthy fruit can be a problem for some. It's a fact that too much stevia can be super sweet and leave an unpleasant aftertaste as well. The trick to Stevia, is to use very little. If we want to stop craving sweets, then we have to stop putting that sweet taste of any kind on our tongues.

It's been a challenge, but also very rewarding, to create healthy life changing products that taste appealing without making them overly sweet and addictive. I am excited that I've been able to do just that with CBD Super Cider, Slender Cider, Green Slender Cider and CBD Super Food. In fact, CBD Super Cider has no Stevia at all. Its delicious taste is thanks to the purity of the pure, organic polyphenol-rich, cherry concentrate and the robust, delicious herbal formula. In fact there are 2.3 GRAMS of herbal blend in each serving of CBD Super Cider.

What you pair your CBD with is as important of the quality of CBD you are putting into your body. Read your labels!

3rd Party Testing

The best way to insure CBD products have the potencies the label claims, is to make sure you can consult their third party testing analysis. A third party analysis should show you the purity of the product—that it has no toxins, microbes, bacteria or metals, it should reveal the full spectrum of cannabinoids, flavonoids and terpenes in the product.

Your Optimal Health

CBD can be taken any time of day, with or without food. As long as you take some of the above factors into consideration, it's really exciting to see the health potential in CBD. I do not think it's a miracle drug. After all these years of working with thousands of people to help them to break free from addiction, lose weight and get healthy, mentally, physically and emotionally, I truly believe health is a result of balance. Self-Hypnosis is a form of meditation that brings balance through connecting to the deeper mind and heart and retraining the habitual thought patterns (in the subconscious). CBD brings balance to the body, mind and emotions because it's a compound that the body recognizes, to bring homeostasis to all its systems. At the same time, the only way to insure optimal health, over time, is to create a balanced lifestyle that includes a life of purpose, including meaningful service, loving, close relationships, deep relaxation, enough sleep, physical exercise and a balanced diet. I do not advocate being on any particular diet—rather eating a simple, healthy diet with whole, real, clean unprocessed food—eaten in a balanced way. To help put an out of whack body-mind back in balance, I highly recommend you embark on a two week mega-nutrition cleanse.

With *Easy Sugar Breakup*, remember there is no diet. The other day I was being interviewed for a national TV news story that was documenting the success of my program, and it struck me when two of my clients who had lost massive amounts of weight with my program (50 pounds and 140 pounds) each said the same thing to the anchor woman who was interviewing them: "I get to eat all the foods I love that make me happy." I love that because I feel the same way. When you change the way you think about food, your criteria for what you put in your mouth changes. You no longer feel deprived because you "can't have pancakes with maple syrup even once a week (like "everyone else does")! That's because you no longer care what "everyone else gets to eat" and you solely base your food choices on how great you want your body to run and feel.

The key to success is make your healthy food taste great. Enjoy every bite! In the next chapter, I am going to show you how to prepare healthy food so it tastes fabulous! I hope you'll thoroughly enjoy experimenting with my easy sugar breakup recipes in the next chapter.

As we've discussed in this past chapter, one of the greatest benefits of CBD is the fact that it puts your body back into balance. To help you maintain inner equilibrium, the recipes you're about to discover are designed to help you eat in a balanced way. Additionally, to assist you in putting an out of whack body-mind back in balance, I highly recommend you take a look at gently cleansing your system.

To do that, I invite you to embark on a magnificent two week cleanse that will help to rid your body of harmful toxins that have been dragging you down. But first, take a look at some of the wonderful recipes you can begin to use as you retrain your body to eat healthfully, while enjoying every bite, and eliminating those trigger foods that have caused you to succumb to cravings.

10. Sugar Cancelling Recipes

With all the contradictory information about what foods are healthy and what foods aren't healthy, you may feel confused and wonder, "What should I eat?"

If I were to give you a diet, unfortunately, it would feel like every other diet—something to rebel against. Not consciously, of course. In the beginning, most likely you would read over the whole diet and get excited. This is something you are going to stick with, you would assure yourself. But the problem is, subconsciously, the minute you go on a diet, you are simply waiting to go off it. The subconscious mind does not want to feel deprived. Remember the job of the subconscious mind is to seek pleasure and avoid pain.

Therefore, the only way to break free from unhealthy cravings permanently or if you are overweight, to keep extra weight off for the long haul, is to change the types of foods you desire. There are two ways to do this and I recommend that you do them both, simultaneously.

One way to do that is with powerful self-hypnosis techniques, by changing your own personal associations with food. For example, instead of picturing ice cream as a treat and something to look forward to, or a way to soothe yourself or bond with others, you can remind yourself that you have the choice to see ice-cream (or any other food or substance) differently.

When you look at ice cream, you can see it as a rich, disgusting, sugary substance, that was created in a laboratory with chemicals, by a greedy, manipulative, billion dollar food industry, for the sole purpose of keeping you—and the rest of humanity—in a prison, addicted. That may seem a bit strong and negative, but to me, it's all about achieving the goal of weakening desire for a harmful substance.

Even if ice-cream isn't bad for some people, it's probably "bad" for you if you are reading this book. In other words, one man's meat is literally another man's poison. It's true that some people can really eat foods like cookies and ice cream in moderation. Those people really wouldn't need to use a technique like the one I'm describing to turn themselves off to those foods. In other words, if it's not a problem, you don't have to fix it.

But if you are craving rich, sugary foods, then there are two ways to stop it. One is by changing your mental associations with those foods by applying self hypnosis strategies, and the other is to physically change your cravings by making your body more alkaline, and eating healthy foods, in balance, including pure protein, throughout the day. Small amounts of protein at a time are fine—but if you really want to be free, you'll most likely discover that animal protein is a necessary staple. The sugar cancelling recipes in this chapter will physically help you to shift your cravings. The reality is that the key to not wanting sugar—or any substance—is to simply remove it from your life.

It's no different than making your breakup with the old boyfriend/girlfriend permanent. When you keep hanging on to the relationship, you really can never move on. But as soon as you cut that person off completely, you can begin a new life.

No matter how attached you are right now to sugar, or any substance, you have the ability to live very happily without it. I honestly never thought I could go a day without ice cream, let alone decades, but when I realized that my sugar/

carb addiction had taken over my life, I knew I had to make an important decision.

I looked into the future with the realization that I was at a juncture; you are also at that same fork in the road this very moment. The issue is which way do we want our lives to go? I knew the road of addiction all too well. Yes, you can cover it up, hide it, and still have success in your life, but at the end of the day, you are left facing the fact that you're an addict. The other choice, which is freedom, seemed like the only viable choice to me. And the only way to get free, I realized, was to have a complete sugar and junky carb break-up (you don't have to give up all carbs—just the empty calorie ones.)

Breaking up isn't that hard when you change the way you see that person—or in this case, food. You can train your mind to see through the enticing smells, alluring tastes, and pretty packaging that the food and alcohol industry sets in front of us. You can look beyond the emotional connections that advertisers attach to their products and edibles.

Instead, you can look at food and drink and ask yourself, "How is this food/drink/substance going to make me feel?" Fast forward in time to that moment, whether it's in 5 minutes, 5 hours or 5 days, where you regret what you ate or drank because you feel gross. Take a mental snapshot of that moment and attach it to the food in front of you. Practicing that strategy can be the secret to quelling desire for harmful foods/substances.

At the same time, you want to follow simple eating principles to bring your body into balance. Balance is the key to success. Your body gets into balance by eating foods that are rich in nutrients. When you get into the habit of choosing foods based on the nutrition and blood sugar balancing components in those items you are eating (rather than just the taste on the tongue that will dissolve in seconds), you can begin to be free from cravings, physically.

Remember to eat according to the Food Map that you created in Chapter Two. You are not on a diet. You are however, remembering that every food has a vibration that either lifts you up or brings you down, and that's especially true with the combinations of foods you eat.

Pitfalls to Avoid

One of the biggest mistakes I see people make is black or white thinking. Carbs aren't bad—please don't become carb-phobic. When you try to avoid all carbs, you are likely to create a feeling of deprivation. You'll notice that my Sugar Cancelling Recipes have carbohydrates also because all carbs are not equal. The goal is to select whole, real, clean, unprocessed food that burns slowly in your body, and satiates (not stimulates) hunger.

Remember, it's best to avoid categorizing yourself and food as "good" "bad" "right" "wrong." Instead, I encourage you to select foods based on how they are likely to make you feel. So ice cream, for example, is not "bad." Maybe your kids or husband can eat ice cream in moderation. But for you, if it's a trigger, then you may choose to avoid ice cream, because you don't like how it makes you feel after you eat it (tired, addicted, etc.)

Now you may argue that you love ice cream because you feel great when you eat it. That may be true, which is why you always want to use that "fast forward in your mind" technique to remember the actual impact ice cream (or any other substance) is having on your life. In any breakup, there are positive memories. But if you really want to be free, you have to focus on the reasons why you are no longer going to tolerate the pain of the relationship (in this case, your relationship with food.)

Lift your mind and look towards the future you want and deserve—happiness, peace, health and freedom. As you gaze forward in time, always remember the alternative possibility. If you keep eating foods that are harmful to you, or that perpetuate addiction, where will you be in 5 months or 5 years? It's always good to be aware of your choices and your inner power to create a destiny that will be fulfilling for you. The key question is, 'is a moment's "pleasure" worth sabotaging ultimate fulfillment?'

The Secret to Ending Physical Cravings

On a physical level the key is, don't let yourself get too hungry. Eat enough protein. You don't have to have large amounts at a time, but small amounts of protein throughout the day can make a huge difference. Protein balances your blood sugar. Carbs and healthy fats satiate. That's why you want to balance protein, healthy fat and healthy complex carbohydrates throughout the day. Do not be afraid of fat. At one time, we were told that fat creates fat. Ultimately, researchers corrected that notion by informing us of the huge difference between harmful fat and the healthy Omega-3 oils that the body needs. Extra virgin olive oil, avocado and flax seed oil are all examples of healthy fats.

If you start your day with oatmeal, for example, enjoy your morning carbohydrate, but be very careful to balance your food intake by eating mostly protein with salad and veggies the rest of the day. Be mindful, when you are eating, of the effect your meal is having on your body.

You'll notice in my recipes that I do use healthy fat, and even some cheese at times. That's because it's essential that your healthy food tastes great. This way you won't ever feel deprived, no matter what the people around you are eating. If your food choices are too bland, you run the risk of being sucked in by processed food again. I recommend that you incorporate the least amount of healthy fat and complex carbs needed to make your food enjoyable.

At night if I'm hungry, I find that cooking up just a couple of tablespoons of anti-biotic and hormone free ground beef with some cabbage or Brussels sprouts is exactly what I need to ward off hunger and satiate. If I were to eat a carb, it would have to be complex, like a small amount of sweet potato or potato. Do pay attention, however. If you choose carbs—even the healthiest carbs, notice if they are they increasing your appetite. It's very possible that they are, especially if you aren't combining with protein.

Listen to your body. It's amazing how protein in small amounts really does help you to avoid wanting more carbs.

Trust Your Inner Wisdom

Another trap I see my clients fall into until they gain new awareness is the idea of choosing foods based on what they read about them. Let's say you are online and you read about all the benefits to eating a certain fruit. Pay attention to how your body actually responds to the fruit you are eating. The criteria for choosing a food needs to be more than just, "Is it a healthy food?" Of course, you only want to eat healthy foods, but you also want to make sure that the foods you choose are best for you. If you are a carb/sugar addict it's likely that even healthy forms of sweetness are triggers for you. The solution? Be very mindful when eating any sweet foods, even healthy ones and always balance with pure protein. Your goal is to avoid tipping the scales, and creating extreme hunger or appetite, from being in an out of balance state.

I'm excited to share my *Easy Sugar Breakup* recipes with you. After awhile you'll intuitively know what foods work best together to keep you completely satiated and energized. If you know a certain ingredient is weakening for you, like dairy, wheat or soy, feel free to substitute it with something else. You can also take some of the recipes and combine them.

Be creative and create your own healthy combinations. Remember that, like it or not, for carb/sugar addicts like you and me, small amounts of high quality animal protein is most likely our best medicine, to balance the blood sugar. Especially if you are selecting one of my recipes with a high complex carb content, make sure to balance your meal with some protein. Most importantly, have fun! The road to health can be a most exciting adventure!

Cottage Cheese Pancakes

Makes Twelve 3" pancakes

Ingredients
¼ cup whole wheat flour or rolled oats
½ cup cottage cheese
2 cage-free eggs
1/8 tsp. sea salt
5 tbs and 1 tsp. milk or pure coconut milk
Optional: almond butter, peanut butter

Directions
1. In a blender, combine flour (or oats), cottage cheese, eggs and sea salt, until smooth.
2. Add milk or coconut milk.
3. Lightly grease a skillet or griddle.
4. Drop spoonful of batter onto griddle and cook at medium high heat on both sides.
5. May eat plain or with a spread of almond butter or peanut butter (or an additional sunny side up egg.)

Breakfast Porridge with an Egg

Serves 4

Ingredients
1 cup warm water
2 tbsp. plain yogurt, kefir or buttermilk
1 cup rolled or cracked oats
½ tsp. sea salt
1 cup water
2 tsp. organic coconut oil
4 eggs
1 tbsp. ground flax seeds
1 tbsp. ground chia seeds

Directions
1. Mix yogurt, kefir or buttermilk with the warm water.
2. Mix oats and soak at least 7 hours, preferably overnight even longer.
3. The next morning, bring one cup of salted water to a boil.
4. Add soaked oats, reduce heat, cover and simmer 2-3 minutes.
5. Meanwhile, heat coconut oil in the skillet.
6. Add eggs without stirring for sunny side up eggs.
7. Spoon oatmeal out into bowls.
8. Sprinkle each bowl of oats with chia and flax seeds and top with one egg.

Non-Dairy Zucchini Cream Soup

Serves 4

Ingredients

1 tb extra virgin olive oil
1 small onion, peeled and chopped
3-4 medium zucchini, chopped
6 cups water or vegetable stock with no sweetener
½ cup oatmeal or rolled oats
½ tsp. sea salt
2 tbs chopped parsley

Directions

1. Heat the oil in a large soup pot. Add the onions and sauté over medium heat.
2. Add zucchini and sauté 2-3 additional minutes
3. Add water, then oats and sea salt, stirring constantly.
4. Bring to a boil. Reduce heat. Simmer 15 minutes.
5. Transfer to a blender and puree. Strain. Add chopped parsley. Serve.

Ginger-broiled Flounder with Red Cabbage and Couscous

Serves 4

Ingredients
3 lbs. fresh flounder or cod
2 tbsp. no-alcohol soy sauce (e.g. Ohsawa Organic Nama Shoyu)
2 tbsp. water
2 tbsp. sesame oil
1 tsp. freshly grated ginger
½ head red cabbage
½ bunch arugula, cut up
½ cup chopped celery
1 ½ tsp. sea salt

Dressing
Juice of one whole squeezed lemon
1 tbsp. no-alcohol soy sauce (e.g. Ohsawa Organic Nama Shoyu)
2 tbsp. extra virgin olive oil

Directions
1. Wash and dry the fish filets and place in a glass baking dish.
2. In a bowl, mix soy sauce, water, sesame oil and grated ginger.
3. Pour over the fish and marinate for at least 30 minutes. Preheat broiler.
4. While fish is marinating, shred the cabbage very fine.
5. Sprinkle with salt, mix well and allow to stand 30 minutes.

6. When the cabbage is ready, rinse salt, drain
    and squeeze out any excess water.
7. Add chopped arugula and celery to red cabbage.
8. Mix lemon juice, soy sauce and olive oil and
    sprinkle lightly on red cabbage and toss.
9. Broil the marinated fish until done.
    Serve with red cabbage.

Avocado with Lemon-Soy Dressing

Ingredients
One avocado
Juice from one fresh squeezed lemon
Spray Braggs Liquid Amino Acid

Directions
1. Cut avocado in half and remove pit.
2. Scoop out flesh with a spoon and slice avocado.
3. Pour juice from lemon on avocado
4. Spray with Braggs Liquid Amino Acids

Cheesy Baked Potatoes Stuffed with Turkey and Cauliflower

Serves 4

Ingredients
2 large baked potatoes
1 lbs. organic ground turkey
2 medium tomatoes cut up
1 tsp. sea salt
1 Tbsp. extra virgin olive oil
2 cups cauliflower, cut up
2/3 cup shredded cheddar cheese

Directions
1. Wash potatoes and prick with a knife in several places.
2. Bake at 400 degrees for 45 minutes, or until soft.
3. On the stovetop, cook ground turkey in a skillet. Add chopped tomatoes and ½ tsp. sea salt.
4. Place cooked turkey and tomatoes in a bowl.
5. Add olive oil to the skillet. Turn heat to medium and add cauliflower pieces. Add ½ tsp sea salt. Cook 8 minutes.
6. When potatoes are done, cut potatoes in half and place cauliflower and turkey-tomato mixture onto potatoes halves.
7. Add shredded cheddar cheese and serve.

Salmon Filet Salad

Ingredients
8 oz. Salmon filet
Olive oil spray
Sea salt to taste
1 bag cut organic romaine
1 oz. cut up red cabbage
1/3 bag broccoli slaw
1 oz. shredded beets
6-7 raw dry roasted pecans
2 tbsp. crumbled blue cheese
2 tbsp. organic flax seed oil
1 tbsp. organic raw apple cider vinegar
½ tsp. Slender Cider (available at http://slendercider.com)
½ tsp. sea salt
½ tsp. dried cilantro
½ tsp. dried dill weed
optional: 2 figs, cut up

Directions
1. Preheat oven to 350 degrees.
2. Place salmon in a glass baking dish. Spray with olive oil and grind a little fresh salt on the fish.
3. Bake for 15 minutes.
4. In a large bowl, mix romaine, cabbage, broccoli slaw, shredded beets, nuts and cheese.
5. In a glass jar, with a tight fitting lid, mix flax seed oil, apple cider vinegar, Slender Cider, sea salt and herbs. Shake jar well.
6. Put dressing on salad and mix well.
7. Add salmon on top. Serve salad and salmon.

Ginger Almond Chicken with Barley, Sunflower Seed & Brown Rice Pilaf

4 Servings

Ingredients
1 cup brown rice, uncooked
½ cup barley, uncooked
½ cup raw sunflower seeds
3 cups water
½ tsp sea salt
3 cloves garlic, minced
1 Tbsp. minced fresh ginger root
2 Tbsp. sesame oil
1 Tbsp. alcohol-free soy sauce (e.g. Ohsawa Organic Nama Shoyu) or Braggs Liquid Amino Acids
4 hormone-free, antibiotic-free, chicken breasts
3 Tbsp. olive oil
1 leek, cut up
1 cup slivered almonds
1 cup snow peas

Directions
1. In saucepan, place brown rice, barley, sunflower seeds and water. Add sea salt.
2. Bring water to a boil and simmer 45 minutes, or until all water is absorbed and rice and barley are soft. Add small amounts of water as needed, if pilaf is sticking to pan or not cooked through. Using a pressure cooker will cut cooking time in half.
3. Mix the minced garlic (you may use a garlic press), cut-up ginger, sesame oil and soy sauce/Braggs Amino Acids, together.

4. Cut the chicken into one-inch pieces. Marinate the chicken pieces in the sesame-garlic-ginger mixture.

5. Heat the olive oil in a hot skillet, on the stovetop. Add the leeks, snow peas and almonds.

6. Cook 2-3 minutes until leeks are translucent and snow peas are bright green.

7. Remove from skillet and place vegetables with almonds on a serving dish.

8. Place the marinated chicken pieces in the hot skillet and cook throughout (5 minutes or so).

9. Add the chicken pieces to the snow peas, leeks and almonds. Serve over brown rice-barley-sunflower seed pilaf.

Tuna Burgers

Serves 4-6

Ingredients
1 large can of tuna, not drained
2 cage-free or organic eggs, slightly beaten
1 small onion chopped
1 tb fresh lemon (juice from half a lemon)
1 tb fresh parsley, chopped
1 ½ cups oat bran
¼ tsp sea salt
Pepper, to taste
1-2 tbs extra virgin olive oil
Alfalfa sprouts, salad greens or baked yams

Directions
1. Mix tuna, eggs, oat bran, onion, lemon juice, parsley and sea salt together
2. Shape into 5-6 patties.
3. Using a griddle pan or skillet on the stove, heat olive oil and cook tuna burgers on each side until browned.
4. Serve with salad greens and alfalfa sprouts or baked yams

Chicken and Vegetable Quesadillas with Cashew Non-dairy Sour Cream

Serves 4-6

Ingredients
1 tbsp. extra virgin olive oil
4 scallions, cut up
3 mushrooms, thinly sliced
1 diced sweet red bell pepper
Rotisserie chicken with the skin removed, cut up
One 15 oz. can of organic black beans, drained
½ cup fresh, chopped cilantro
½ tsp. sea salt
1-2 cups fresh, washed, cut arugula
8 whole wheat tortillas (read labels – look
for wraps with no oil or sweeteners)
1 avocado, sliced

Sauce
2 cups raw cashews, soaked in water for at least 4 hours
¼ cups water
2 tbsp. extra virgin olive oil
2 tbsp. organic, raw apple cider vinegar
Juice from half a lemon, fresh squeezed
2 minced cloves garlic
1 tsp. sea salt

Directions
1. In a skillet, heat up the oil, and add scallions, mushrooms and red pepper. Cook 1-2 minutes.
2. Add chicken, beans and cilantro and heat through. Transfer mixture to a bowl.

3. To make sauce: blend in a high-speed blender cashews, water, oil, apple cider vinegar, lemon, garlic and sea salt. Set aside.
4. Spray skillet with olive oil. Place tortilla in the skillet and let brown 1 minute or so.
5. Fill half the tortilla with the chicken-bean-vegetable mixture. Add arugula pieces.
6. Top with cashew-garlic sauce, fold over other half of tortilla and flip to cook the other side.
7. Do this one by one for each of the tortillas. Cut and serve with slices of avocado.
8. Put remainder of cashew sauce/ dressing in the refrigerator.

Buckwheat Crepes with Almond Butter

Makes 15 crepes

Ingredients
3 eggs
½ cup milk or pure coconut milk (no
sweeteners or chemicals)
¾ cup plain yogurt
½ cup buckwheat flour
¼ cup whole wheat flour
1 tb organic butter
Almond Butter

Directions
1. In a bowl, beat eggs until thick. Stir in milk and
   yogurt. Sift in buckwheat and whole wheat flour.
2. Let a little of the butter melt in a skillet.
3. Pour in some of the crepe batter. Cook on
   medium heat, flipping crepes over so they
   are lightly browned on each side.
4. Serve with a tsp of almond butter.

Green Pea Salad with Chicken

2 servings

Ingredients
8 oz. cooked hormone-free chicken
thighs or breasts, cut up
10 oz. package frozen peas, thawed and drained
¼ cup slivered almonds
½ cup chopped celery
1 small onion, chopped
¼ cup chopped green pepper
2-3 tbsp. plain non-fat yogurt

Directions
1. Mix all ingredients together.
2. Chill before serving.

Chicken Vegetable Miso Soup

Serves 4

Ingredients

3-4 pieces of wakame seaweed
1 tsp. butter
4 scallions, chopped
1 clove garlic, minced
4 cups water
3 carrots, sliced
½ cup shredded cabbage
2 stalks celery, chopped
1 cup cooked diced chicken
4 Tbsp. miso paste

Directions

1. Soak wakame seaweed in a small bowl in cold water for 2-3 minutes.
2. In a large pot, melt the butter on low heat. Add the scallions and garlic and sauté until soft.
3. Add the water. Put soaked wakame, carrots, cabbage, celery and chicken in the pot.
4. Bring close to a boil. Cover the pot and turn the heat off. Let vegetables simmer.
5. Put the miso paste in a small bowl. Ladle a small amount of the soup broth and pour over miso and mix.
6. Put the miso broth into the large soup pot and stir.
7. Do not let the miso boil as this destroys the enzymes and changes the taste. Serve

Beef and Garlic Broccoli

Serves 4

Ingredients
1 lb. grass-fed or organic ground beef (may use ground turkey)
Sea salt
1 medium onion, peeled and chopped
½ cup water
1 bunch broccoli, washed and chopped
1 clove garlic
1 tbsp. sesame seeds
Sea salt to taste
½ cup fresh grated mozzarella

Directions
1. Form beef into hamburger patties. Sprinkle with sea salt.
2. Place in large skillet. Turn heat on high. Brown on both sides.
3. Turn heat down. Add onions. Cover. Simmer approximately 10 minutes, until burgers are done.
4. Put water into a medium sauce pan and add the broccoli and garlic.
5. Cover, lower heat and let steam for 4 minutes.
6. Uncover and put the stems on the bottom, florets on top.
7. Steam another 2 minutes. Season with sea salt. Add shredded mozzarella cheese.
8. Dry the sesame seeds by putting in a dry hot skillet and letting them brown for a few minutes. Watch carefully. Sprinkle the dry roasted sesame seeds over the broccoli.
9. Serve broccoli with hamburgers.

Quick and Easy Eggplant with Beef or Turkey

4 Servings

Ingredients

2 medium eggplants or 1 large eggplant,
peeled and sliced lengthwise
Extra virgin olive oil in a spray bottle
Braggs Liquid Amino Acids in a spray bottle
1 lbs. grass-fed hormone-free ground beef or turkey
½ tsp. sea salt
1 leek, cut up
1 clove garlic, minced

Directions:

1. Spray each slice of eggplant lightly with olive oil and Braggs Liquid Amino Acid
2. Place on outdoor grill or on baking sheet under your broiler
3. Grill or broil until lightly brown. Turn over and grill or broil the other side (approximately 2-4 minutes each side)
4. While the eggplant is cooking, brown beef in skillet on high heat. Turn heat down and while simmering, add leek, sea salt and garlic.
5. When meat is thoroughly cooked, and leek and garlic are cooked through, drain.
6. Take eggplant off the grill and cut into one-inch strips.
7. Serve with beef.

Tuna with Vegetables

Serves 2

Ingredients

1/8 cup organic apple cider vinegar
Splash Slender Cider (available at http://SlenderCider.com)
½ tsp. Dijon mustard
1½ tsp. fresh basil
1/3 cup organic flax seed oil
2 cups fresh, washed and cut up organic spinach
1 cup cut-up organic lettuce
1 small carrot shredded
½ cup alfalfa sprouts
½ cup chopped sweet red pepper
6 ½ oz. tuna, water-packed and drained
¼ cup crumbled feta cheese

Directions

1. Blend the apple cider vinegar, Slender Cider, Dijon mustard and basil in a small blender. Add the flax seed oil and blend until smooth.
2. In a large bowl, add the spinach and lettuce.
3. Arrange carrot, alfalfa sprouts, pepper, tuna and cheese on top.
4. Cover with Flax-Dijon dressing to taste. Mix well and serve.

Turkey, Potato and Spinach Casserole

Serves 4-6

Ingredients
4 baking potatoes
1 lb. hormone-free ground turkey meat
1 small can tomato sauce
1 tbsp. extra virgin olive oil
1 ½ tsp dried cilantro
½ cup chopped scallions
4 cups fresh spinach leaves
8 oz. shredded cheddar cheese

Directions
1. Preheat oven to 375 degrees.
2. Wash potatoes and prick 2-3 times with a fork.
3. Bake for up to one hour, until soft and done.
4. In a skillet, cook up the ground turkey. Add tomato sauce.
5. Remove from stove and set aside.
6. In a skillet, heat the olive oil.
7. Add cilantro and scallions. Cook 2 minutes. Add spinach. Mix thoroughly and cook about a minute.
8. Combine turkey mixture with scallions and spinach.
9. Take potatoes out of the oven when they are cooked through.
10. Cut potatoes open. Stuff with meat and spinach mixture.
11. Sprinkle with cheddar cheese. Put back in oven just long enough to let the cheese melt. Serve immediately.
12. Add sea salt to taste.

Zucchini Crust Pizza

Serves 2-4

Ingredients
4 cups finely grated zucchini (in a blender), liquid squeezed out
1 tbsp. extra virgin olive oil
2 cloves minced garlic
4 tomatoes, finely cut
1 tsp. dried parsley
1 tsp. dried basil
1 tsp. dried oregano
½ tsp. sea salt
½ cup water
1 cup spinach leaves, washed
6 oz. fresh mozzarella cheese, sliced
3 tbsp. grated parmesan cheese
5 tbsp. ground almonds
1 cage-free egg, beaten

Directions
1. Preheat oven to 350 degrees
2. Spread ground zucchini on a baking dish and cook in the oven, 5-7 minutes, remove and cool.
3. To make the sauce, heat the olive oil in a large skillet.
4. Add the garlic, tomatoes, parsley, basil, oregano and sea salt.
5. Add ½ cup water to tomatoes while cooking.
6. Let sauce cook 10-15 minutes.
7. Steam spinach in a small amount of water in a saucepan and put aside.

8. When zucchini has cooled, squeeze out all excess liquid with a cheesecloth.
9. Mix the cooked zucchini with the parmesan cheese and the ground almonds and egg. Add a dash of sea salt. Form the mixture into a large ball for the crust.
10. Spray a baking sheet with olive oil spray.
11. Break the zucchini ball into two balls and pound down to make two round pizza crusts.
12. Preheat oven to 450 degrees
13. Bake the two zucchini pizza crusts until brown (about 15 minutes)
14. Top both crusts with tomato sauce, fresh mozzarella, and spinach.
15. Put back in oven and bake until cheese melts (2-3 minutes longer)

Non-Dairy Creamy Mushroom Barley Chicken Soup

Serves 4

Ingredients
2 cups fresh chicken stock (made by boiling
chicken parts in water, with vegetables)
3 large onions, chopped
2 cloves minced garlic
6 tbsp barley
5 fresh mushrooms, washed and chopped
1 cup diced cooked chicken
¼ cup fresh, chopped parsley
2 tbsp. fresh chopped dill

Directions
1. In a medium sized saucepan, bring
   the chicken stock to a boil.
2. Stir in the onions, garlic and barley. Cover.
3. Reduce heat to low and simmer 45 minutes.
4. Add the mushrooms. Cover and
   simmer 15 more minutes.
5. Add the chicken. Turn off heat.
6. Using a slotted spoon, transfer solids
   from soup into a blender and puree.
7. Return the puree to the liquid in the
   soup. Add dill and parsley.
8. Bring the soup to a boil. Turn off heat and serve.

Chicken Zucchini Casserole

Serves 5-6

Ingredients
8 oz. organic cottage cheese
½ tsp. dried oregano
½ tsp. sea salt
1 tbsp. extra virgin olive oil
1 cup sliced and peeled yellow summer squash
1 green pepper, seeded and coarsely chopped
1 red onion, sliced and separated into rings
3 cups sliced and peeled zucchini
2 sliced fresh tomatoes
1 lb. cooked hormone-free chicken thigh
or breast, cut up into 1-inch pieces

Directions
1. Pre-heat oven to 350 degrees.
2. Oil a large glass baking dish.
3. Mix together cottage cheese with oregano and sea salt.
4. In casserole, layer the vegetables, chicken
   and cottage cheese mixture.
5. Bake for 50-60 minutes and serve.

Healthy Easy Sugar Breakup Desserts

Frozen Banana Pops

Ingredients
4 small, very ripe bananas

Directions
1. Peel bananas and place on wooden sticks.
2. Place bananas in Freezer bags.
3. Place in the freezer until frozen.

Spiced Raisin Squares

Makes 16 servings

Ingredients
1½ cups whole-wheat flour
½ cup cooked brown rice
½ cup raw pecans, chopped and dry roasted in a skillet
1 cup golden raisins, soaked in boiled
water to cover, with soaking water
1½ tsp. baking soda
1½ tsp. cinnamon
½ tsp. ground ginger
¼ tsp. ground nutmeg
1/8 tsp. ground allspice
2 eggs
¼ cup organic coconut oil
Optional: 1 dropper pure liquid Stevia (Use
pure Stevia only, with no Natural Flavors)
1 cup buttermilk
1 tsp. finely grated orange peel

Directions
1. Preheat oven to 350 degrees.
2. In a large bowl, combine the flour, rice,
   pecans and raisins with soaking water.
3. Mix with baking soda, cinnamon,
   ginger, nutmeg and allspice.
4. In another bowl, beat the eggs and add oil (and stevia).
5. Add the buttermilk and orange peel to the egg mixture.
6. Stir together thoroughly.
7. Pour batter into a baking dish.
8. Bake 30-35 minutes or until done.

Carrot and Raisin Loaf

Ingredients
2 cups whole wheat flour
1 tbsp. aluminum-free baking powder
2 cage-free eggs
½ cup organic coconut oil
1 cup shredded carrots
1 cup chopped raw walnuts, dry-roasted in a skillet
¾ cup yellow raisins, soaked in boiled water
to cover, overnight, with soaking water
1 tsp. finely grated lemon peel
Optional: 1 dropper pure liquid Stevia (Use
pure Stevia only, with no Natural Flavors)

Directions
1. Preheat oven to 350 degrees.
2. Combine the flour and baking powder in a large bowl.
3. In a bowl, beat the eggs.
4. Add oil, carrots, walnuts, raisins and lemon peel
    with soaking water, and optional Stevia.
5. Add the wet ingredients to the flour mixture.
6. Transfer the batter to a baking pan or bread pan.
7. Bake at 350 degrees for one hour or until done.

Almond Date Cookies – Gluten Free

Makes 16 cookies

Ingredients
1 cup raw organic almonds
½ cup cut-up dates
½ cup brown rice flour
1 large cage-free egg
1 tsp. pure vanilla extract

Directions
1. Grind ½ cup of the almonds plus dates and the flour in a food processor, until completely fine.
2. Add the egg and vanilla and mix well.
3. Press the mixture into the bottom of a lightly oiled square baking pan.
4. Add tiny drops of water, as necessary, for spreading.
5. With a knife, mark off two inch squares.
6. Press one or two almonds in the center of each square.
7. Bake on the top rack of the oven for 15-20 minutes or until tops of cookies are light brown.
8. Cool. Cut the cookies on the marked lines and remove from pan.

11. The Two-Week Mega-Nutrition Cleanse

Embarking on a Two-Week Mega-Nutrition Cleanse can act as an easy transition to help you make a complete shift in your dietary habits. Although the focus of the cleanse is on drinking fresh, nutrient-filled juices, it does not include fasting. There are many books on the benefits of total juice fasting. However, since I am a strong advocate in the importance of fiber and protein, I find it advantageous to combine fresh, raw vegetable juicing with eating fresh, raw vegetables such as salad and cut-up, shredded, or grated veggies. I find this to be a much more gentle approach. This would include juicing vegetables and eating lots of salads and vegetables with olive oil or flaxseed oil. Aside from these sources of healthy fat, small amounts of animal protein (chicken, fish, or lean meat) are also recommended during this cleanse to keep the level of sugar in your blood steady. This is because your primary goal is to eliminate cravings for sugar and simple, refined carbohydrates, so you don't want to shock your body by upsetting your blood sugar dramatically. Condiments such as freshly minced garlic and herbs can be used for flavoring.

Many of us think in terms of, is a food healthy or not? Instead, it can be more useful to look at a particular food and assess its unique effect on your body as opposed to whether or not it would be universally considered a healthy food. In other words, while the health benefits of meat may be questionable to some, for others it is a food choice that has great value in restoring health.

It may seem contradictory to eat meat during a time when you are cleansing the body of toxins. Surely, we can read a lot about the negative effects of beef, and even chicken, on the body. It is true that meat has a high saturated fat content, and this can have a detrimental effect on the cardiovascular system, according to many studies. However, there is an equal amount of evidence that it is not the animal protein that is the problem, but the high sugar (and fat) content in the processed food that makes up the average American diet that is the real culprit when it comes to the devastating increase in disease and obesity in this country.

Your goal is to purge your system of the need for the insidious chemicals in the foods that you may typically be used to eating—such as store-bought or restaurant-prepared processed food. During the two weeks, when you eat whole, natural foods and fill your body with nutrient-rich (preferably organic) juice from greens and other vegetables, you will begin to free your body from the ill effects of the toxic food from the past. When you keep your blood sugar steady with a regular supply of protein, your system can find equilibrium. After the two weeks, it will be much easier to incorporate complex carbohydrates back into your diet in a balanced way, without the need to revert back to sugar-filled desserts, sauces, or dressings. After two weeks without table salt, small amounts of sea salt to flavor your food can be incredibly satisfying. The hefty amount of sodium inherent in most prepared foods will likely become so much more obvious and distasteful.

A Gift of Health

How you view this two-week period will make a huge difference in the benefit you gain from it. In other words, it is imperative that you do not think of this cleanse as just another diet that you are attempting. Rather, it is helpful to see this cleanse as a gift of health that you are giving to yourself—an opportunity to purify your body of a buildup of toxic substances. When you think that the goal of your cleanse is to break the body's addiction to certain foods and the chemicals in the foods, you can look forward to the freedom of preferring the foods that are best for you.

How to Deal with Physical Withdrawal

Like letting go of every addiction, giving up sweets may leave you with some withdrawal symptoms. The most common symptoms are fatigue, depression, anxiety, nausea, headaches, and gastrointestinal upset. The great news is that these symptoms are short-lived, and when you understand that your body is simply repairing itself and you use the tips in this chapter, you can get through any mild withdrawal stage with ease.

Part of getting through withdrawal is just being patient with yourself and understanding what's happening. Your body needs to begin to cleanse and rejuvenate itself from all the assaults of the past. It has an incredible ability to be resilient and wants to reach a state of homeostasis and health. During the cleanse, it's very important that you treat yourself with gentleness and kindness. As your body cleanses itself, rids itself of toxins, and begins to fill with the nutrients it has been crying out for, you will experience a completely new level of health, energy, and vitality. Take the opportunity to pamper yourself during this two-week period.

- Give yourself some time and space.

- Take warm Epsom salt baths to speed up the cleansing process. The salt will help draw toxins out of your body.

- Go outdoors and get plenty of clean, fresh air and, if possible, find beautiful places in nature where you can sit or lie down, undisturbed.

- Spend time with yourself journaling, drawing, or painting.

- Treat yourself to a therapeutic massage. Massage is a very effective means to remove toxins from the lymph system.

- Regular physical exercise will expedite the release of toxins from your body. Choose a form of exercise that you really enjoy. Try jumping on a trampoline, walking in water, Rollerblading, or playing racquetball. Since you will be taking in less calories, make sure to listen to your body, and do not overdo the physical activity at this time!

- Deep breathing is a wonderful way to purify and energize your bloodstream by carrying revitalizing oxygen to your heart and entire cardiovascular system. This in turn feeds the brain and all the organs and cells of your body. It's a great idea to start practicing

the deep breathing and stretching exercises you
learned in Chapter 5 to facilitate the release of putre-
fied matter from your body.

When you get through the withdrawal stage by drinking fresh
juices and selecting healthy, nutritious raw foods as outlined in
this Two-Week Mega-Nutrition Cleanse, you will slowly begin
to acclimate to a new way of eating. This is not as dramatic
as fasting for a few days and then going back to old, harmful
eating behaviors, or substituting new, unhealthy foods and
liquids in place of the old, which can happen quite easily.

Eliminating the Toxins

You have many organs of elimination, including the skin, kidneys, lungs, and most important, the colon. A healthy colon
is a strong indicator of a healthy body. One way to keep the
colon clean and well is to eat raw, natural foods and to stop
eating before your stomach is full. Another effective means
to maintain a healthy bowel is through drinking fresh vegetable juices. Fresh, raw vegetable juicing is a wonderful aid
to cleansing and rejuvenating your system and will help you
immensely during a withdrawal phase, since it will flood your
body with much-needed nutrients.

Because the fiber has been removed, fresh vegetable juice
is quickly assimilated and digested, with minimal effort from
the digestive system. This gives your body an opportunity to
rest, while the cells, tissues, and organs are saturated with
minerals, vitamins, and essential enzymes. As your body
begins to receive the elements that it needs to thrive, you
will move through any withdrawal stage with ease and soon
return to the state of vibrant health that is your birthright.

Juicing vs. Blending

Recently, one of my clients asked me why it was preferable to juice vegetables and fruits rather than use one of those high speed blenders? That's an excellent question. There are definitely pros and cons to each. As always, I recommend trusting your inner wisdom to know exactly what's best for your body. There is no right or wrong here.

The benefit to pulverizing your vegetables and fruits using a high speed blender is that it keeps the entire plant intact. Therefore you are also getting all the fiber along with the nutrients inherent in the produce. That's a very good thing, especially when you are drinking plenty of water along with your blended veggies.

The reason I am recommending juicing vegetables with this particular two week cleanse, is because when you put your veggies through the juicer, because you are eliminating the fiber, it's possible to consume a much greater quantity of nutrient-rich vegetables. In other words, you can juice an entire head of celery, loaded with essential enzymes, minerals and vitamins such as folate, potassium, vitamin B6, vitamin C and vitamin K, and flood your body with those essential nutrients. By contrast, when you put the celery in a high speed blender, though you'll get the added benefit of fiber, it's most likely that you will only be able to consume a much smaller portion of the celery. So ultimately, your body is getting many more nutrients when you juice.

The other issue is taste. Unless you happen to like pulp, most people prefer the delicious, pure, clean taste of veggies that have been run through the juicer. There is no need to add any sweetener. Since we are always subconsciously seeking pleasure and avoiding pain, if you don't like the foods you are consuming, it won't be long before you abandon the entire regime. That's just the way the brain is wired. That's why it's essential to select foods and activities to maintain your highest level of health, that make sense and feel pleasurable to you, both consciously and subconsciously. Simply put, you are much more likely to make a positive choice, like juicing, a habit, when you enjoy it.

If it turns out that you absolutely prefer blending your veggies, there is certainly no harm in it, and blending, too, is very beneficial. Again, I want to caution you about adding sweeteners of any kind to your drinks. I highly recommend against it. So if the only way that you can enjoy your smoothies and blended drinks is with a lot of fruit or/and added sweetener, please consider making a different choice, especially if your goal is to be free of food cravings and addiction.

Blended drinks and vegetable juices, however, are perfect beverages to add either CBD Super Cider, CBD Super Food and/or Slender Cider to. None of these herbal concentrates are particularly sweet, but they taste very pleasant and will add to your drink a whole lot of nutrition as well as alkalizing, energizing and balancing components.

Discovering Food Sensitivities

This two-week cleanse is also a wonderful way to become aware of any possible food sensitivities that may be causing you to have an intense desire for certain items. Often we crave the very foods that are toxic to our system, spawning food sensitivities and extreme hunger. Intuitively, we may assume that we wouldn't crave a food if it was harmful for us, but that is not the case. Often, the items that we are most sensitive to—even ones that some consider to be healthy such as soy, wheat, or dairy—are actually creating unpleasant symptoms for ourselves. For example, we may feel tired a lot and seek a glass of milk or a cookie made with dairy to bring ourselves energy. Although the short-term goal is attained, upon further examination, along with food elimination, we may discover that it was the cream or milk itself that was the culprit. In this case, we may stop consuming dairy and notice a dramatic increase in our energy level.

When you embark on the Two-Week Mega-Nutrition Cleanse, you will cleanse your system of any potential allergens because you will be consuming an assortment of vegetables, with small amounts of various types of protein that you will be rotating. Why rotate your proteins? Because if you are sensitive to any particular protein—let's say, chicken, for example—it will be much easier to identify the culprit if you are not eating the same thing every day.

For the duration of the cleanse, you'll have no grains, starchy vegetables such as corn or potatoes, condiments, dairy, or soy.

This way, when you reintroduce foods from the "Foods to Eat in Moderation" category in Chapter 8, you'll quickly be able to discover any that are potentially harmful to you. Eliminating a food for a two-week period of time and then reintroducing it is a terrific way to determine which foods cause you to be symptomatic. Typically, if a food causes you to experience an adverse reaction, such as indigestion, a headache, irritability, or a drop in energy level, it will be remarkably more noticeable following a period of abstaining from that item or category of food. For example, if after being on the cleanse for two weeks, you eat a piece of Swiss cheese and react, you may be sensitive to that particular cheese or to the entire category of dairy foods. It becomes easier to pinpoint those foods that are causing you harm. Also, following the cleanse, it will become so much easier to walk away from these allergens, as the cleanse will break your compulsive tendency and free you from the pull toward those foods you used to crave.

What Is the Two-Week Mega-Nutrition Cleanse?

During the two weeks of the cleanse you will be drinking fresh vegetable juices that you will prepare at home daily. You will select only foods from the vegetable (water-rich foods), healthy fat, and animal protein categories found in Chapter 8, "High-Nutrition Eating."

During this two-week cleansing period, it's best to eat raw vegetables as much as possible. However, if you have trouble digesting raw veggies, or have an aversion to them, it's fine to eat cooked vegetables. You can simply steam them, or sauté them very lightly in extra virgin olive oil. Either cooking method works very well with collard greens, broccoli, kale, cabbage, or brussel sprouts.

You will eat small amounts of animal protein regularly, rotating different types of fish, chicken, and meat (or eggs) daily for the duration of the two-week cleanse. In other words, it's OK to have chicken with your vegetables one day, the next day perhaps you will select eggs to go with your veggies, another day flounder, for example, and the next day may be halibut.

It's OK to use some of the cold-pressed oils, in moderation, during your cleanse. That would include grape seed oil, extra virgin olive oil, and flaxseed oil. If you have a hard time eating vegetables plain, adding just a little cold-pressed extra virgin olive oil may give your cooked vegetables just the flavor they need. The only other condiments you will use during the cleanse are fresh herbs such as garlic, parsley, cilantro, and dill. Feel free to use them liberally so you can fully enjoy what you are eating.

Preparing for Your Cleanse

To get ready for your Two-Week Mega-Nutrition Cleanse, as much as you can, eliminate processed foods from your house. This includes sauces, prepackaged foods, and condiments that you may use regularly. You may be astonished to discover the high level of saturated fat, table salt, sugar, and other chemicals that you are ingesting regularly. If you live with other people and it's not possible to discard these items, at the very minimum get rid of your favorite processed foods so there will be less temptation to succumb to.

During this two-week cleanse you will avoid all the foods in the lists "Foods to Eliminate" and "Foods to Eat in Moderation" in Chapter 8. I do suggest that you avoid all dairy, including any kind of cheese or butter, during the initial two-week cleanse, although down the road, cheese and even a small amount of butter may become foods that you can eat in moderation. Also, avoid starches, whole-grains, all nuts and nut butters, seeds, soy or salt, during your cleanse.

If your mind starts making assumptions about how deprived your life will feel because you'll *never* be able to eat the foods you *love*, remind yourself very gently that you are taking this one day at a time. If there is a food you feel that you absolutely must have, let yourself know that if you still feel this strongly after the cleanse, you will give yourself permission to eat this food. This is not an exercise in deprivation, but rather an opportunity to take your life to a new level of health and freedom from food, or any substance, addiction.

You'll need to purchase a fresh vegetable juicer. I like the Champion Juicer, although it is a bit of a hassle to keep it clean. You'll want to look for an excellent quality juicer that can handle juicing fresh vegetable greens, including wheatgrass, which is a wonderful internal cleanser. It is well worth the investment to buy a high-quality juicer that can withstand extended use and succeed in juicing various types of vegetables. Another way to get your daily Organic Wheatgrass, Organic Spirulina and Organic Barley Grass intake, is by sipping Green Slender Cider. Slender Cider is a liquid herbal concentrate of 11 organic, therapeutic herbs, with or without greens, in a base of raw, organic apple cider vinegar (available at RenasOrganic.com).

By preparing and drinking fresh vegetable juices daily, you are helping to speed up your body's cleansing process. Take a look at the list of vegetables in Chapter 8, as well as some of the possible juice combinations you'll read about later in this chapter, and then make a list of all the vegetables that you would like to use. You may even think of some other vegetables that are not on those lists.

When you leave the house, make sure that you have an adequate supply of food and drink, so that you can keep your blood sugar steady. Although the vegetable juice is a wonderful way to fill your body with vitamins, minerals, and nutrients, the fact that it is void of fiber can affect your blood sugar. That's why it will be necessary for you to eat plenty of fiber-rich foods, such as whole vegetables, combined with some protein, to keep from getting too hungry.

Remember, the purpose of your two-week cleanse is to purge your body of the perceived need for sugary, processed, empty-calorie foods, release toxins that perpetuate cravings, track down and eliminate any food sensitivities, and begin to fill your cells with vitamins, minerals, and phytochemicals that build health. You want to take extra care to keep your blood sugar steady and avoid any dramatic dips by incorporating fiber into your diet. Aside from the vegetables that you will be eating, if you are prone to constipation, I highly recommend a fiber supplement, such as psyllium seed. This will not only help to detoxify the colon and release toxins, but, like all fiber, will slow the rate at which the food you eat is released into the bloodstream.

Additionally, taking fiber supplements is one way to encourage yourself to stay hydrated, since it is the water you drink that causes the psyllium to expand in your intestines and do the work of improving your body's elimination. Fiber supplements are available at your health food store or online. A word of caution—be sure to avoid harsh fiber supplements, such as those with Senna. In addition to psyllium seed, I highly recommend Rena's Organic CBD Super Food. It's very gentle yet it has all the benefits of 250 mg of water soluble, organic CBD plus 24 additional super foods, greens and herbs, each of which is a wonderful source of fiber. The following is a list of what you will need to begin your cleanse:

- A high-quality vegetable juicer

- A stainless steel thermos (stainless steel won't distort the flavor)

- Containers to take your vegetables and protein with you

- A cooler bag to put the containers in

- A selection of vegetables for juicing

- A selection of salad and vegetables to eat, either raw or slightly cooked

- A good fiber supplement

- Plenty of protein on hand: salmon and other kinds of fish, eggs, fresh roasted turkey breast (do not use cold cuts), and slices of beef brisket, lamb chops, pot roast, or steak to nibble on (Avoid canned meats at this time.)

- Fresh cold-pressed oils, such as extra virgin olive oil and flax-seed oil

- Lots of fresh spring or distilled water (You may want to invest in an at-home water distiller.)

Recommended supplements:

Slender Cider and/or CBD Super Cider – The herbs in both Slender Cider and CBD Super Cider are great for digestion, increasing metabolism and energy naturally and healthfully, and assimilating. Both are in a base of organic apple cider vinegar, which is very alkalizing. The more alkaline your body is, the less you crave sweet and salty foods. Neither product has any sugar or artificial sweeteners. CBD Super Cider is one of the only CBD products on the market to have USDA organic certification. The Concentrated formula contains 400 mg. full spectrum CBD, along with 2.3 grams Cannabinoid-rich herbs, per serving, and polyphenol-rich organic cherry concentrate (no flavors).

CBD Super Food is a nutrient-rich energy powder blend with 250 mg. water soluble CBD, to bring balance to your body. The CBD is a wonderful aid to bring homeostasis to your whole body.

Fresh Juicing

There is a big difference between fresh, raw juicing and drinking juice from a bottle or can. Not only do many of these drinks have harmful additives, but they also have been heated in the canning and pasteurization process. In addition, you have absolutely no way of knowing how long the can or bottle has been sitting on a shelf. When you make your own fresh vegetable juice, you can be assured that the nutrients your body is craving are intact. Fresh vegetable juices are free from the harmful table salt found in abundance in the canned variety.

It's best to drink vegetable juice immediately after you juice it. The nutritional value is highest when the juice has just been extracted from the vegetables. However, if it is not possible for you to make the juice several times a day and drink it fresh, take some along in a high-quality stainless steel thermos. Also have a cooler bag and some containers or ziplock bags so that you can take your vegetables and salads with you, as well as your protein.

Making Your Selections

Next, go to your local health food store, farmer's market, or natural foods market and look for organic, fresh produce. Buy a variety of vegetables, especially greens, for both juicing and munching on. It's OK to use some sweet vegetables, but you'll want the majority of your selections to be a variety of nutrient-rich greens, to avoid perpetuating sugar cravings in your system.

I recommend collards, kale, mustard greens, cabbage, spinach, parsley, and broccoli. Avoid vegetables that you know you don't like. If you've always hated cauliflower, for example, don't force yourself to eat it. There are plenty of options that you are sure to enjoy, instead. I can't emphasize enough the importance of listening to your body.

Perhaps the only greens you like are salad greens. If so, stock up on plenty of spring mix, arugula, and romaine. Fresh sprouts are a wonderful option, as the live food is filled with health-promoting nutrients. Grated veggies such as broccoli slaw or red cabbage add a delicious crunch to your salads. This is about finding pleasure in healthy foods, so select the ones that you can start out liking the best. Yes, your taste for food will change and you are likely to start enjoying healthier foods more and more, but respect your process and begin with the vegetables that you feel most drawn to.

When you buy beets and carrots for juicing, if you can, select the ones that have the greens still attached to them. When you choose the whole vegetable, you are getting more nutrients. If you like, buy some garlic and ginger to add a bit of zest to your drink. Cucumbers and celery are wonderful cooling foods that will enliven your juicing experience. (Do not include the celery leaves, as they will make your juice taste bitter.)

Even though fruit is filled with life-promoting nutrients, minerals, and vitamins, it has a very high sugar content. Sensitive individuals can react to too much fruit in the same way they would react to a candy bar, being barraged with a host of symptoms brought on by a spike in blood sugar followed by an episode of hypoglycemia or low blood sugar, as a result of insulin being over-secreted.

As you learned earlier, when considering your selections, the only issue is not whether a food is healthy, but even more important, how is your unique system going to react to it? Over time, you'll become more and more adept at determining that before you eat the offending foods. It is for this reason that I personally not only limit my fruit intake but also do not add any fruit to my fresh juice.

Remember that it's best to select foods that are low in natural sugar and high in fiber, which slows down the release of sugar, such as fresh green vegetables. Even some vegetables, such as carrots and beets, can be very sweet tasting as well as detoxifying, so again be careful and pay attention to the effect of the foods you are eating on your body. If you choose to use apples and other fruits such as strawberries, grapes, grapefruit, or the sweeter vegetables in your juice, use them sparingly, due to their high natural sugar content, and experiment with adding just enough of these high-sugar foods to make the juice palatable. Keep your approach gentle.

After you have purchased your vegetable (and possibly fruit) selections, make sure to wash them carefully when you get home, particularly if they are not organic. Though, I do encourage you to get only organic produce if at all possible. Dry the vegetables by spinning them and store them in your refrigerator in ziplock bags. To increase their shelf life, remove any excess air from the plastic bag.

Fresh, Pure Water

Water is essential to life, and drinking a gallon of water per day is an integral component of the Two-Week Mega-Nutrition Cleanse. Almost 70 percent of your body is composed of water. How much water do you drink each day? In order for your body to function at an optimal level, you need to make sure that it is properly hydrated. Water helps fill you up so you aren't as hungry. It also helps to relieve food cravings, regulate the body's temperature, remove wastes, and transport oxygen and nutrients to the cells. It increases the absorption of nutrients, aids in proper digestion, and helps generate cellular energy.

The high level of sodium inherent in all processed food, including commercial salad dressing and soups, is a major cause of dehydration. When we consume a lot of sodium, we are taxing the kidneys, because they begin working overtime. Also, since the water that we do have in our system needs to be available to dilute the sodium concentration, it is not free to perform its other necessary functions.

We may not even realize that we are dehydrated. Often we reach for food instead of filling our body with what it is really crying out for—water. Being dehydrated on a regular basis can cause you to overeat and eat the wrong foods.

Often people are afraid to drink water for fear of becoming bloated, but in reality the opposite is true. The less we drink, the more the body retains water. Drinking pure water helps to increase energy, sharpen your mental and physical performance; reduce stress, depression, anxiety, and headaches; and promote weight loss.

I recommend that you start drinking at least sixty-four ounces of water every day (or half your body weight in ounces). Wake up in the morning and drink two or three full glasses upon arising. Continue drinking throughout the day. If you don't like the taste of water, it can be helpful to experiment with different types of water. For example, when I switched to distilled water, I found myself able to drink far greater quantities than when I was drinking filtered water. My body began to crave the pure and clean taste of the water.

If you decide to go that route, you may choose to buy yourself a water distiller so you can make distilled water daily, in the convenience of your home. The other obvious advantage of distilled water is that all the chemicals that pollute tap, bottled, or well water are removed. Much of our drinking water is contaminated with pollutants such as pesticides, fertilizers, herbicides, toxic waste from landfills, and acid rain. Using distilled water eliminates the risk of drinking water from the tap or a bottle, since bottled water is not highly regulated. According to the Federal Council on Environmental Quality, U.S. drinking water contains more than 2,100 toxic chemicals that can cause cancer, and yet the EPA only regulates 87 of them. The advantage of drinking distilled rather than filtered water is that filters can easily collect bacteria if they aren't changed often enough—and it's often difficult to determine how frequently to change the filter.

Another trick to making drinking water more palatable is to add Slender Cider Concentrate to your water. For many people, including myself, Slender Cider makes drinking water a lot more like second nature. Drinking boiled water with fresh squeezed lemon offers a unique water drinking experience, as well.

Selecting more whole, unprocessed, water-rich foods along with increasing the amount of water you drink every day will help you to stay hydrated. Aside from oxygen, water is the body's most vital element.

The Cleanse

Here are the basic rules of the cleanse:

1. During the two-week cleanse, you may eat as many vegetables and drink as much fresh vegetable juice as you like.

2. Begin each day of your daily cleanse with a fiber supplement (as needed) and at least one or two full glasses of spring or distilled water, upon arising.

3. Make your first batch of vegetable juice in the morning, using the recipes in the next section. Have some protein and vegetables with your juice for each meal and snack. As healthful as the fresh vegetable juice is, it still can cause your blood sugar levels to spike and then plummet if it is not tempered with fiber and protein. I recommend drinking 4 –8 ounces of juice each time.

4. During your cleanse, make sure to eat every two hours to prevent hunger. It's fine to just eat a small amount. Try to go by your body's own hunger signals. Don't worry if at first you can't tell when you are physically hungry. As you follow the program it will get easier and easier for you to determine your level of physical hunger (as opposed to appetite).

5. Drink lots of water during the day. A gallon of water is not too much to drink in a day when you are cleansing your system. Remember that water is a wonderful way to relieve the body of toxins it has been carrying.

6. If you have a tendency to get constipated, remember to take your fiber supplement and/or Rena's Organic CBD Super Food, daily.

Daily Protein Choices

- Hard-boiled eggs (organic, or hormone and antibiotic free)

- Omelet with spinach, prepared with olive oil or vegetable broth

- Broiled halibut, grouper, flounder, or salmon, drizzled with olive oil

- Fresh roasted turkey (Purchase a turkey breast at the grocery store and follow the cooking instructions on the label. Use olive oil instead of butter, if necessary.)

- Broiled, baked or grilled chicken

- Grilled steak or lamb

Rotate your proteins so you can more easily spot potential food sensitivities. If you have eggs on Monday, select fish on Tuesday, beef on Wednesday, and turkey on Thursday, for example. Have one type of protein per day.

Breakfast

- A glass of fresh vegetable juice

- Animal protein; e.g., 2 eggs

Lunch

- Prepare a big salad with your favorite greens, such as spring mix, arugula, romaine, and chopped raw vegetables such as broccoli slaw, red cabbage, beets, or sprouts.

- Top the salad with just enough flaxseed or olive oil to wet the leaves and approximately 6 ounces of the animal protein of your choice.

- Enjoy your meal with a glass of fresh vegetable juice.

Morning and Afternoon Snacks

- Midmorning and midafternoon, have some celery or cucumber sticks with a small piece of chicken or meat or an apple with a slice of cheese (if you have not eliminated dairy).

Dinner

- Steamed vegetables such as broccoli, cauliflower, zucchini, yellow squash, kale, collards, or red chard. You may drizzle with olive oil and/or herbs such as dill or cilantro.

- Approximately six ounces protein, such as fish, poultry, or meat.

- A glass of fresh vegetable juice.

Evening Snack Options

- One thin slice of beef with a raw carrot.

- One thin slice of turkey breast with a raw cucumber.

- Cold salmon with two leaves romaine.

- A glass of vegetable juice with a small piece of animal protein.

Daily Juicing Suggestions

The instructions for each of the juice recipes below are the same. Wash each of the vegetables and cut to fit through the mouth of the juicer. Turn the juicer on and feed them through one at a time. When using smaller vegetables, such as ginger slices or garlic cloves, you can wrap them in the leaves of your green vegetables, then feed the leaves through the mouth of the juicer. Drink juice while it's fresh, or if necessary, place in a stainless steel thermos and save for a time when it's convenient to drink. For the greatest therapeutic benefit, extract your juice in small batches and drink it immediately after juicing since the longer the juice sits, the more nutrients are lost.

Here are two juicing recipes for each of the fourteen days of your cleanse. Feel free to experiment with your own combinations. Adjust the carrot, apple, and beet portion to meet your needs. For example, if you find yourself experiencing symptoms of hypoglycemia, such as extreme hunger, fatigue, mood swings, cravings, irritability, dizziness, or anxiety, you may want to cut back on the sweet vegetables and fruits.

Day 1

Drink 1
- 2 kale leaves
- 1 handful spinach
- 2 stalks celery
- 1 wedge cabbage
- 1 handful parsley
- 2 carrots (or add carrots to taste)

Drink 2
- ½ small fennel bulb
- 2 carrots
- ¼ beet
- 2 collard leaves

Day 2

Drink 3
- 1 wedge red or green cabbage
- 4 stalks celery

Drink 4
- 6 sprigs watercress
- 6 sprigs parsley
- 3 carrots (or less if palatable)
- 5 broccoli florets

Day 3

Drink 5
- ¼ to ½ head cauliflower
- 4 carrots
- 2 celery stalks

Drink 6
- ½ head broccoli (florets and stalks)
- 2 carrots
- ½ apple

Day 4

Drink 7
- 2 pieces Swiss chard (both the leaf and the stem)
- 1 or 2 carrots to taste
- 3 ounces alfalfa sprouts

Drink 8
- 3 beet greens
- 1 handful spinach
- 1 handful parsley
- 2 carrots
- ½ apple (seeds removed)

Day 5

Drink 9
- 2 endive leaves
- 1 handful parsley
- 4 carrots
- 2 stalks celery

Drink 10
- 2 apples (seeds removed)
- 2 stalks celery
- 1 beet
- 1 bunch watercress
- ½ lemon

Day 6

Drink 11
- 2 cucumbers
- 1 apple (seeds removed)
- 1 yellow squash
- 1 zucchini

Drink 12
- 1 handful collard greens
- 4 carrots (to taste)
- 1 stalk celery

Day 7

Drink 13
- 3 radishes
- 3 ounces alfalfa or radish sprouts
- ¼ beet
- 1 parsnip
- 1 cucumber
- 1 leaf romaine

Drink 14
- 1 bunch dandelion leaves
- ½ head broccoli (stems and florets)
- 1 celery stalk
- 1 cucumber
- 2 carrots

Day 8

Drink 15
- 1 handful kale leaves
- 1 parsnip
- 1 green pepper
- 1 or 2 carrots

Drink 16
- 1 bunch red Swiss chard
- 1 bunch dandelion greens
- 3 or 4 carrots

Day 9

Drink 17
- 1 bunch spinach
- 1 apple (seeds removed)

Drink 18
- 6 romaine leaves
- 2 stalks celery
- ½ cucumber

Day 10

Drink 19
- ½ head broccoli
- 3 brussels sprouts
- 2 carrots
- 1 apple

Drink 20
- 2 kale leaves
- ¼ beet
- Beet greens
- 3 stalks celery
- ½ cucumber

Day 11

Drink 21
- 8 romaine leaves
- 1 parsnip
- 1 carrot

Drink 22
- 1 red pepper
- 4 ounces alfalfa sprouts
- 3 carrots
- 1 handful watercress

Day 12

Drink 23
- 2 kale leaves
- 1 handful parsley
- 1 stalk celery
- 1 cucumber

Drink 24
- 3 Swiss chard leaves
- ¼ beet
- 3 sprigs watercress
- 2 carrots

Day 13

Drink 25
- 2 romaine leaves
- 1 clove garlic
- 1 handful parsley
- 1 handful cilantro
- 3 carrots
- ½ apple (seeds removed)

Drink 26
- 3 or 4 spinach leaves
- 5 dandelion leaves
- 2 kale leaves
- 3 carrots
- Fresh mint or basil

Day 14

Drink 27
- 2 cucumbers
- 1 stalk celery
- 2 or 3 carrots

Drink 28
- 1 wedge red cabbage
- 2 stalks celery
- 2 carrots
- ½ cucumber

Other Optional Juicing Ideas

Drink 29
- 3 stalks asparagus
- 1 handful spinach
- ½ cucumber
- 3 carrots

Drink 30
- 3 stalks asparagus
- 2 brussel sprouts
- 1 handful mustard greens
- 1 handful watercress
- 4 carrots

Drink 31
- 2 kale leaves
- 2 celery stalks
- 1 handful parsley
- 3 carrots
- 1 apple (seeds removed)

Drink 32
- ½ green or red pepper
- 2 celery stalks
- 1 carrot
- 1 cucumber

Drink 33

- 4 radishes
- 3 ounces alfalfa or radish sprouts
- 1 handful parsley
- 3 carrots

Drink 34

- 1 2-inch slice jicama
- 2 stalks celery
- 2 carrots

Drink 35

- 2 Swiss chard leaves
- 1 handful parsley
- 1 ¼-inch fresh gingerroot
- ½ apple (seeds removed)

Drink 36

- 5 broccoli florets
- ½ beet with greens
- ½ apple (seeds removed)
- 1 handful parsley

Drink 37

- 6 sprigs watercress
- 6 sprigs parsley
- 1 wedge green cabbage
- 2 carrots

Tips for a Successful Cleanse

During the next two weeks, remind yourself that being slightly empty (but not hungry) is a great way to insure health. It allows you to breathe more deeply, which you will discover is a strong key to health and freedom from addiction. For optimal health, your stomach should be filled with one-third air, one-third water, and one-third food.

Before bed, after you've treated yourself to a nice, warm bath, enjoy some soothing music, and then take fifteen minutes to sit or lie quietly and practice your deep breathing exercises. Make it part of your routine to incorporate deep breathing every day, since as you learned in Chapter 5, a vital component to health is lots of oxygen.

Remember to chew your food slowly and savor the delicious flavors. Digestion begins in the mouth, so take time to chew each bite thoroughly. When you begin to eat foods in their more natural state, as you are doing in this Two-Week Mega-Nutrition Cleanse, you can begin to appreciate the flavors that are inherent in the foods from the earth, without being masked by all the sugar and chemical-filled sauces we so quickly become accustomed to. Relish the nutrients that you are taking in, and feel your own personal connection to the earth as you allow yourself to be nourished by all the wonderful food that the earth provides for you.

Connect with the vital life force that is flowing through you. Eating in this simple way for a two-week period will not only help you to cleanse your system physically, but also connect you more deeply with your deeper self and the gift of life. If you haven't had a chance to be in nature during the day (which I highly recommend), or even if you have, spend a few moments before you drift off to sleep imagining your favorite place out in the woods or at the ocean shore hearing the waves lapping onto the beach.

Smell the freshness of the mountain air, in your imagination, and take in the beauty of a fragrant rose. Take pleasure in the uniqueness of who you are, and feel your connection to all of life. Give thanks for the food that has nourished you on this day, and for the strength to follow through on a goal that is so important to you—gaining freedom from compulsion around food or harmful substances. This is a type of self-hypnosis that can help you to access your greatest resources as you program yourself for success.

Listen to Your Body

If at any time during the cleanse, you feel weak or out of balance, tune in to what you are needing. You may need to incorporate a small amount of whole-grain, like brown rice or sweet potato. Though the goal is to purify and eliminate any potential triggers, if you are feeling that you need more balance with what you are eating, pay attention. Even if you shorten the cleanse to one week, or even three days, you are doing a great service to your overall health. The important thing is to transition off the cleanse gently so that you can maintain all the benefits.

After the Cleanse

Clearly, the whole point of the Two-Week Mega-Nutrition Cleanse is to begin a new way of life. After the two-week period, you can begin to introduce complex carbohydrates from the list in Chapter 8, but slowly. Don't go off the first morning and have a big whole-grain bagel. Yes, that is surely better than a conventional bagel, but it still poses the danger of triggering binge eating.

Remember what you have learned about the importance of balance. Continue to make vegetables (and vegetable juice if you care to continue juicing), salads, protein, and healthy fat the mainstay of your diet, and incorporate the carbohydrates slowly. For example, at breakfast, have half a whole-grain bagel, drizzled with a dash of olive oil, with your spinach omelet. The oil is high in calories, but it will help to decrease the glycemic value of the bagel, causing it to be burned up as fuel a little more slowly, thereby avoiding triggering a low blood sugar reaction.

Congratulations! You are on your way to a life filled with more energy and vitality. As you continue to incorporate water-rich, unprocessed food into your diet more and more, you will naturally begin to prefer those foods that are sustaining your life! It will only get easier to stay on track with your new, positive eating habits as you combine mega-nutrition eating with breaking free from inner states that have led to food cravings in the past. Trust yourself and embrace the new eating habits that are enhancing your quality of life. Honor the part of you that sincerely longs to not only be free from obsessions about food, but also to really value and care for yourself—and have your actions reflect that. You are worth it!

Conclusion: Enjoying the Benefits of a Craving-Free Life

Now it's time to celebrate! When it comes to food cravings, food addiction, addiction in general, and health, ultimately each of us needs to discover our own way. There is no one eating and lifestyle plan that works for everyone. However, the fact is when we eliminate certain foods or substances from our diet, we no longer crave them. The desire vanishes. For many of us, this is a symbol of true freedom.

It is heartbreaking to see so many people trapped by their own desire—concerned that they would be deprived if they didn't get to eat certain foods. And yet, as you now know, the very foods many of us eat perpetuate the feeling of wanting them. When we begin, instead, to select foods that nourish the body—delicious, fresh vegetables, greens, fruits, whole-grains, nuts, seeds, extra virgin olive oil, flaxseed oil, and high-quality protein—we no longer miss the junk we used to eat as a substitute for real food. We begin to feel healthier and in control of our life and eating habits, fully enjoying the freedom of eating to live rather than living to eat.

Taking Control of Your Life

Obviously, it would be ideal if we could shift the whole food paradigm so that processed food and drink were no longer the norm. And certainly that is a worthy goal to work toward. But until these changes happen on a broader scale, it is essential that you make the necessary alterations in your own diet and your personal way of relating to food. You may be right in assuming that there is no way to avoid chemical exposure in your foods, or even in the air you breathe. Though that is true, you certainly can make the decision to limit your processed food intake, switch to drinking distilled water, add a few key nutrients such as organic full spectrum, medical grade CBD for overall balancing of all your bodily systems and incorporate deep breathing and exercise into your daily regime. Even though you cannot prevent yourself from having emotional reactions, you can learn to use the Break-Your-Craving-State Technique to eliminate their harmful effects on you and stay more connected to your deeper, wiser, more resourceful self.

As you continue to adopt healthful behaviors as components to a richer existence, you may be surprised and delighted by the control that you have in your life. Just changing your thoughts alone can bring about a radical shift in your behaviors and preferences. For example, if you typically used to drink soda, every time you think about reaching for a diet cola, don't think of the taste (if you like it)! Instead, go directly to imagining the chemicals in these drinks and the incredible toll consumption of these beverages may have on your health.

When you begin to perceive that the sweet taste is a momentary pleasure that is costing you a huge price, it will become a lot easier to just let that go. To expedite that process, focus on the price you are paying rather than on any perceived pleasure. If you experience headaches frequently, for example, tune in to the suffering you endure and imagine that your attachment to soft drinks (or whatever your weakness, whether it be chips, wine, beer, pot, pills or candy) is the culprit. Even if you are unsure whether that is true, by making that assumption you are helping yourself to break a habit that can only be having a negative effect on your entire system.

Use the headaches (or the weight gain, irritable bowel, PMS, depression, and so on) as a source of motivation to change the pattern of reaching for soda throughout the day to give you energy or reward yourself. Find new, positive behaviors that can fulfill you. What a treat it would be to find a quiet place in the middle of the day, lie down, and practice fifteen minutes of deep breathing instead.

Learn to be conscious about what you are putting into your mouth. Be gentle with yourself, as this requires practice, particularly if you are used to eating anything you want, whenever you want, mindlessly. The first step is to become aware that you pay a high price for continuing with this habit and make and affirm your decision to change your ways.

Rating Your Desire and Progress

Throughout the day, do the following exercise with foods that hold a strong pull for you.

. . . .

EXERCISE: DO I REALLY WANT THIS FOOD?

When tempted by foods that are potentially harmful to you, imagine those foods in front of you and ask yourself, how much do I want this food? Give the food a rating on a scale from 1 to 10. What is your level of desire for this food, with 10 being a must have and 1 being not at all? Then ask yourself what you have to do in order to bring the number down one notch.

Perhaps you need to imagine the food you are craving mixed with a food that you despise, causing the flavors to be inseparable. Or you may need to visualize yourself blowing up so that you can barely move because you've eaten so much of that food it has literally made you sick. Do whatever it takes internally to bring the number on the scale down to the point where you no longer desire the food. For some of my clients, simply imagining all the chemicals hidden in the food that would be ingested into their bodies is enough to turn that desire off. Use your imagination to help you achieve what you desire most—total freedom from food addiction.

Just the other day I was working with a woman named Shelly, on Skype. Shelly had reached out to me to help her with weight loss. I was so impressed with how she was already using hypnotic principles to quit eating sugar. She said that for years every time she was in the grocery store checkout, she would reach for a candy bar, mindlessly.

But then she watched a show on Addiction and heard the expert say that addiction to any substance can only be changed by changing the way you think. Shelly thought to herself, "Why wouldn't this work for food addiction?" and decided to change the way she thought about sweets. She distracted herself when she was in the checkout line, from that day forward by looking at the magazines. In fact, that's how she found me! She was flipping through a magazine at her grocery store checkout, when she came upon my client, who was on the cover of First for Women Magazine, for losing 40 pounds with my Sugar Divorce hypnosis program! Shelly had reached out to me for hypnosis to help her to reprogram her own mind to not want sugar anymore. And it worked!

Another way to help yourself move along from a less desirable to a more productive state is to rate your experience.

. . . .

EXERCISE: MOVING UP THE PROGRESS SCALE

Imagine that your peak weight and health state is rated at a 10, using a scale of 1 to 10. Create that peak state in your mind's eye to make it as real as possible. Use all your senses. Imagine your clothes feeling loose. Imagine yourself enjoying the delicious taste of foods that are light and healthy. See yourself vibrant, happy, and fully alive. If you have trouble imagining yourself in such a positive light, find a picture of someone you imagine to be in great shape and superimpose your face on that photo. Imagine yourself walking briskly, enjoying the feeling of a gentle breeze on your skin and relishing the solid earth beneath your feet. The image you create may be a memory of yourself from an earlier time in your life, or you may create a brand-new image of yourself that represents a possible future.

After you've done that, look at the other end of the scale and imagine what a 1 would be. A 1 (one) may be someone who exhibits no self-care—perhaps the person doesn't even brush his or her teeth. Perhaps a 1 would be someone whose diet consists of only refined sugar, simple, processed carbohydrates, and salty, high-fat food, eating all day long and barely doing any activity at all.

Now, as you gaze at this continuum, where do you find yourself on a scale of 1 to 10? Write down your answer, and also write down your reason for placing yourself at that particular location on the scale.

Perhaps you would place yourself at a 3. Your rationale for doing so is that you do currently walk about ten minutes a day—though not consistently. Also, you eat fairly healthfully and consciously during the day, selecting low-fat foods and some fruits and vegetables. It's only at night that you binge on sweets. Take a moment to congratulate yourself for being as high as a 3 on the scale, and not lower.

It can be astonishing to discover that even when we are faced with difficulty in our life, taking a moment to feel gratitude that it's as good as it is—and not worse (we could be a 1 on the scale) helps increase the probability that we will continue in the desired direction. Unfortunately, the reverse is also true. When we develop the mental habit of berating ourselves, being hard on ourselves, and not feeling grateful for any progress we are making, no matter how minute, we set ourselves up for failure. Gratitude and praise to ourselves and to life— even with the hardships and setbacks—helps give us the strength and impetus to move forward.

Now ask yourself what you need to do to move forward one digit on the scale. Don't set the bar too high. If you rate yourself on the scale in this moment, how can you progress one notch to a level 4? Finally, take a moment to once more imagine yourself at a 10 and savor the fabulous feelings, knowing that this is the goal you are moving toward.

Committing to these small shifts in your habits can propel you into the forward-moving momentum you've been longing for. Moving up the scale in increments is a way for you to be gentle with yourself as you hold the inner vision of your peak weight state.

Keep Setting Your Intention

Every day reconnect with your intention to change your life for the better and to free yourself from food or any other addiction. Continue with the practice of allowing your intention to emanate and spring forth from the deepest place inside of you as opposed to being a mere rote uttering on your tongue. To help increase your sincerity, remember to place your hand on your upper chest—your metaphorical heart—breathe into this place, and bow your head down to your chest, which will help to quiet your chattering mind. This simple act of placing your hand on your chest sends a signal to the analytical, judging part of your mind that you are taking a break from it and making contact with your deep subconscious mind—and your essence.

Let your head rest in the bounty of your heart, and connect into what you truly desire for your life: health, peace, happiness, love, and freedom. When you set your intention to take the higher road in your life, you are setting in motion, within the field of infinite possibilities, a new potential for the course of your life. You are in essence creating a new destiny to be free from the old, unproductive eating habits of the past. You are saying yes to making new choices in your life that support what your heart truly longs for. You are literally reprogramming your subconscious mind to prefer healthier, life-sustaining food over rich, processed food that numbs you, dulls your senses, and compromises your health.

By getting in touch with a wiser, more expansive part of yourself and setting your intention from this place, you are connecting with your greatest source of power, which has the capacity to blast through the voice of fear and expose its inherent powerlessness. You come to see that it is possible to be free from compulsion around food and transform your life into one of radiance, health, and happiness.

Accessing Your Greater Strength Daily

Remember that your deep, wise heart knows exactly what is right and true for you. It is your source of strength, personal power, and knowledge of the truth—and is accessible when you open your awareness more fully. It's here that you will continue to stay in touch with your true longing to love and honor your body and make the best choices for yourself. Sure, you still may notice the temptation of the cookies, but you will have a much deeper awareness that the cookies— no matter how tasty—would not sustain you over time and therefore would be a poor choice.

As you practice the Break-Your-Craving-State Technique regularly, you'll more and more know that the desire for these cookies is simply covering over a greater need within. With this larger perspective, it's much easier to walk away from the cookies, without having to engage much willpower, and fulfill your deeper needs in a much more direct way.

When you are in touch with the core of your being, you are also able to access the inner strength and wisdom necessary to approach your life in a new way. With this greater clarity, you can ask yourself, "What am I needing right now? How can I give that to myself? Am I physically hungry in this moment? What food would sustain me? What am I feeling in this moment? Can I simply be with this feeling, make space around it, and breathe into it? Can I drop all judgments and expectations about what

I am supposed to be experiencing or what I would prefer to be feeling right now? Who am I, beyond this momentary thought or feeling? Is this thought just a habit?"

Even with this new understanding, know that it's natural to fall back into the illusion that you are your thinking, analytical mind. You'll need to remind yourself frequently that behind your conscious mind is the home of your true self—the part of you that not only wants to live in freedom and happiness, but also knows how to do so. Each time you recall your greater nature, you have the potential to get in touch with your larger purpose for being alive.

You may begin to ask yourself questions such as, "What is my highest choice in the bigger picture of my life?" and "How can I best serve myself right now? If I in fact experienced the true gift of my life—my essence—what choice would I make in this moment? Even if I am not feeling any deeper part of myself in this moment, what would happen if I pretended or acted as if there were a wiser part of myself present here to guide me?" If you get stuck when you make these inner inquiries, use the image of a wise teacher, Divine Love that unites us all, or compassionate friend here with you in the moment, watching you without judgment, loving you and guiding you.

As you explore your own nature more deeply, you'll begin to gain a tangible understanding that overeating and indulging in unhealthy, addictive behavior limits your ability to step into the highest potential for your life. At the level of your deeper heart and soul, you can get a real sense of the profound presence of love and higher intelligence that exists within and the vital role your life holds in this world. The preciousness inside you and the need to honor and respect the body that houses your spirit and makes your life possible becomes apparent.

When you live from this place, you are guided to eat the foods that are of the highest choice for you—whole, natural, unprocessed, water-rich foods. You don't have to be phobic about eating fat anymore because you'll discover first hand that a diet that includes enough healthy fat, within the context of a balanced food plan, can ward off hunger and compulsion to eat processed food.

The need for addictive, overly sweet, processed foods begins to drop away. When we finally access our greater potential and break free for good from the painful food addiction that at one time had us completely trapped, there is an indescribable sense of relief and a strong knowing that we will never again return to the old way of being. You can finally trust yourself! This is both my own personal experience and the experience of thousands of people who have attended my hospital-based hypnosis program for weight control. You can escape from the old conditioning that is creating suffering in your life and open to the amazing possibility of a life filled with health, energy, inner peace, and vitality.

Accepting What's True

The key to entering this deeper realm is awareness and detachment. In this book you have learned how to open to a greater awareness of what you are truly experiencing on every level. In other words, rather than blocking out painful emotions, you feel them and acknowledge them, as you have learned to do. This does not mean that you need to act them out or suppress them, but simply recognize that they are there because this is what is true, in this moment. This requires a commitment to being honest with yourself.

So if, in this moment, you are feeling dark and depressed or hopeless, instead of running away from those feelings you begin to explore them by feeling the sensations in your body with a sense of detached curiosity, as if you were just a witness. The sooner you let go of the story line (by questioning your assumptions rather than just accepting all your thoughts as true, and looking at the situation through a wider lens) while at the same time simply allowing yourself to feel the feeling in your body—and the underlying need—the faster you will be able to transcend the pain that you are in and find a more complete truth.

This is quite different from masking the pain by pretending that it doesn't exist or bingeing on candy or alcohol or popping pills to distract yourself. It takes courage to move into, rather than away from, painful feelings, but it is truly the way to freedom, if you are willing to go through them. If you remove the label of "painful" or "depressed," and instead concentrate solely on the physical sensation, without judgment or criticism, it becomes a lot easier.

So let's say you just completed your Two-Week Mega-Nutrition Cleanse and have been eating well for a few months now. You are meeting your husband at a party tonight after work. Your kids are with a babysitter, and you are looking forward to a lovely evening with your spouse. In your mind, you are very excited about spending time with him, and you have the whole evening planned—you'll leave the party together after a short time and stroll through the city, enjoying the crisp autumn air. Unfortunately, not only is your husband an hour late to meet you while barely mumbling an apology, but he becomes completely engrossed in conversations with other people and shows no signs of wanting to leave the party with you even though you've asked him a couple of times.

You feel yourself reacting because your need for control is not being filled. You realize that you cannot control your husband's choices, and yet you feel a familiar sinking feeling and assume that the evening's plans are ruined. Perhaps you notice your urge to hover around the hors d'oeuvre table for most of the evening, but instead make the effort to socialize with some of the guests you are drawn to. You enjoy your conversations, but still feel a sense of disappointment over your husband's choices. Eventually, you leave the party much later than you wanted to, with a sense of sadness and loss.

Now, rather than dwell on the details of the scenario, trying to figure out if you are right or wrong, justified or overreacting, the cause of the problem or the effect, I am suggesting that for true healing to occur, the first step is for you to really notice and honor what you are feeling, without minimizing it or blowing it up. You may simply let the whole thing go and enjoy the time with your husband when you finally do get to have that cherished time to be together, understanding that he was taking advantage of the social gathering as an opportunity to connect with potential clients. Give yourself credit for making the wise decision to enjoy the time that you do have together.

However, so you don't end up suppressing feelings with a binge later on, it's important for you to be honest about what is true for you. If you notice lingering sensations after the incident, give yourself some space to process whatever is coming up for you. When you have a chance to be alone with yourself, notice if there is a lump in your throat. If you want to cry, do not stifle the urge. If you feel anger, be with it, and keep looking deeper for the emotion behind the anger. Often anger points to a deeper emotion such as fear or sadness. Ask yourself, "What am I angry about?" Keep traveling within to the deeper issue that your emotions are pointing to. Notice if there is a tightness in your solar plexus. Maybe you want to run off and have a bottle of wine. Feel the impulse, but do not act on it. Describe to yourself what you are feeling. Perhaps your statement to yourself is this: "I'll never be happy. I'll never feel loved. I am all alone." Perhaps when you travel even deeper within, you find that there is a part of you in a great deal of pain. This may be a feeling that remains from earlier in your life—perhaps when you were very young.

Take some deep breaths into the physical sensations in your body from which these conclusions emanate. Affirm to yourself, "I love you. You deserve to be happy. I am loveable. I am beautiful. I am worthy of love," just as you did in the mirror exercise in Chapter 3. Keep saying this to yourself no matter what your reaction. Repeating the mirror exercise is a way for you to heal any old feelings you may have that are standing in the way of your happiness and your freedom from compulsion around food. As you practice being with what you are feeling in the moment, you will become more aware of what is actually true for you. It may not be nice, and it may not be pretty, but it is what is real for you at that particular time. As you accept your current experience, rather than suppress or cover it up, you are creating an opportunity to heal the recurring feelings that in the past you have blocked out with addictive behaviors. Perhaps as you stay with the physical sensations in your body you will become aware that the feelings you are wanting to escape from are familiar. The way out of food addiction—and all addiction—is to have the strength and courage to go through the blocks that are keeping you from experiencing what is real for you in any given moment.

This strength can only be found in the deeper layers of yourself. Within your core, you can find the power, inspiration, and determination necessary to break through the limitations of the past. Prior to discovering your true essential nature, you may have overly identified with the parts of yourself that are struggling or are less evolved. By connecting into your core self, through the heart, you can begin to tap into your deeper wisdom that can guide you.

Imprinting New Positive Images

Remember that one of the best ways to get a tangible sense that there is a deeper power for good and for transformation inside yourself is to use symbolism and imagery. The following exercise will help you.

. . . .

EXERCISE: INCREASING YOUR INTERNAL RESOURCES

Take a moment to ask yourself what you need right now. Perhaps you need strength, or gentleness, beauty, or playfulness. Now allow an image to come to you that symbolizes this quality. If you need strength, you may see an image of a fierce lion. Feel the strength in the animal and drink it in, deep into your being. A beautiful, strong oak tree with huge, solid roots plunging into the ground may come into your awareness. Feel the solidity, beauty, and grounding of this tree. Allow the strength of the animal or tree to seep into your cells so that you can embody this strength.

If you are craving gentleness, imagine a baby lamb or a soft, loving puppy licking your face. Open to receive these gentle kisses, using all of your senses. Let the child in you experience absolute joy as you imagine a baby's shrieks of delight as it splashes in the bath or plays in the snow. Imprint these images on your heart and etch them into your mind as anchors that can bring you back to the qualities that are your true nature—strength, joy, resilience, and peace.

When you are stuck in painful emotions that you instinctively wish to move away from, resist the urge to disconnect from yourself, and instead breathe into your feelings. Allow yourself to access the strength, gentleness, safety, and beauty within your essence by drawing upon the symbol or image that helps you to connect with this deeper place. Let this place within you—this place of greater intelligence and understanding—beyond the limitations of the mind and personality, fill you with what you truly need.

You can discover what your deeper needs are by being in touch with your feelings. So if you are feeling despair, your deeper need, very likely, is to feel love. The love you are seeking may not be apparent in your outer world at this time. But it also will not be found through food, pills or drink. It can only be accessed through the bounty of your spirit, when you are willing to feel your feelings and surrender them to that which is greater than your small self and greater than the place where the thought formed and the feelings originated.

What's Behind That Feeling?

If you are feeling bored, rather than try to fill yourself up with processed junk food, notice how that habitual action is actually a way of inflicting pain on your being. Instead, sit with your boredom—the sensations in your body—and inquire what the feelings are about. What you are experiencing may be a very important signal from your inner self about a change needed in your life. Perhaps this sensation is a way to nudge you—an urge within yourself to achieve something or contribute in a more focused way to your family, your community, or the world. When you begin to explore the sentiment that you are calling boredom, you may realize that the gift of this feeling is that it prompts you to take a greater action, to walk through a fear that has been holding you back or fulfill a dream that has been struggling to rise from deep in your soul. Rather than mask this feeling with food, you can begin to explore it.

Abraham Maslow was a psychologist who spoke of the hierarchy of human needs. At the very bottom of the scale is our basic need for food, water, clothing, and shelter. As we begin life, these are necessary to sustain our existence in the body. When these needs are fulfilled, the human requirements naturally increase and we proceed to having greater needs such as the need for touch, love, confidence, and security. At the top of Maslow's hierarchy of needs is the need for self-actualization and fulfillment.

As we climb the ladder of life, many of our basic needs are already being filled on a consistent basis. Therefore a yearning for something more is natural and expected. We need to listen to these longings, as they are steering us forward, taking us to the next level in our life. No matter how long you have spent trying to block out the voice of deep wisdom from inside your heart and soul urging you to move forward, take chances, and step into a greater possibility for your life, you cannot get away from it.

The voice of truth only becomes louder and more insistent, and it calls to us in many different ways.

I am sure that you have heard someone who experienced a horrible blow in his or her life—such as grave illness—later claim that it was the best thing that could have happened to him or her. Often we do not begin to pay attention and make necessary changes in the way we live until we are banged over the head or the rug is pulled out from underneath us. You can stop clinging to old routines and familiar habits and patterns and step into your greater potential by choosing to listen to the voice of truth and acting in accordance with it.

Building a New Foundation

Each day that you choose to eat healthfully and simply— selecting whole, unprocessed foods from the earth and balancing your foods—know that you are building a new foundation for yourself. At first, this foundation may feel wobbly, as it is new to you, but every time you make the choice to follow through and select water-rich foods as the mainstay of your diet, eating only the foods that are best for you, in balance, you are adding cement to that foundation. Soon it will be the home that you live in. And though there are sure to be times when you will slip and make mistakes— choices that don't support your deeper intention to live free from food addiction—your new foundation will be there to climb back up on. You will learn to trust yourself more and more and identify with this new way of living and eating as who you really are.

Balance is the key for every meal. Remember your own personal food map that you created in Chapter 2, with the foods that are most harmful to you on the far left, foods that are best for you on the far right, and the moderate choices in the middle. Continue to select foods, as much as possible, from the right side of the spectrum, so that when you eat foods from the middle part of the chart (cheese, whole-grain pasta, and so on) you are not going to begin swinging over too far to the left. When that pendulum starts swinging to the left is when you can feel your whole system tipping over into that familiar food-craving nightmare. It can be very helpful to create a visual image in your mind of this pendulum and how you can keep it stabilized in a balanced state. When your body is in balance, your health and your life feel like they are on an even keel.

The beauty of having completed your two-week cleanse is that you have given your body a jump start toward healthful eating. As you begin to incorporate complex carbohydrates like whole-grains and root vegetables back into your diet, you will probably enjoy them even more than before. Processed, white flour–filled, sugary, empty-calorie, high-fat food will seem revolting to you now that your system knows how good it can feel when it is nourished by pure, healthful food from the earth. Adding just the right amount of medical grade CBD to your diet, can help you to stay balanced mentally, physically and emotionally. Remember what's true, however, with any addiction. Always be aware of the possibility of being sucked back into your old way of life either by sheer habit, laziness, or your environment and the people around you. Make a conscious decision not to let that happen.

Staying on Track

Also keep in mind the concept of momentum. One slipup isn't going to make much difference. But when you allow the voices in your head to convince you that you might as well continue with compulsive behavior since you've already made a mistake, be conscious of what's happening. Don't just go into a numb state and let the past dictate your current mode of behavior. You do have a choice! Turn yourself in the opposite direction, down the road that leads to your ultimate desire for your life: freedom from food addiction. Realize that as soon as you make the decision to turn, you switch the momentum and the direction in which you are headed. It's like you are re-setting the GPS to where you truly want to go. In that moment you are choosing to take your destiny back into your own hands rather than leave it at the whim of your limited, shortsighted ego-mind.

So, let's say you have an "accident" and eat some Fettuccini Alfredo. That's OK—simply go back on the cleanse for a day or so. This will help bring your body back into equilibrium immediately, before your pendulum can really swing to the far left (leading to a full-fledged binge). Otherwise, don't be surprised if you start craving all the old, processed foods you used to eat. Don't beat yourself up about what happened. In fact, enjoy the fact that you got to have the pleasure of such a rich meal. But let it go, and get right back to your new way of eating. The chemicals in food are just as dangerous as any other drug we may get addicted to. In fact, they can be even worse, because it's often difficult for part of us to believe that the foods we used to eat regularly (and all of society is consuming) could really be so harmful when they are so prevalent. The fact that processed fat and sugar–filled food is so common often makes it harder to buy into the reality that the foods we are eating are absolutely chipping away at the quality of our life, if not our lifespan itself.

If the high-fat, high-salt, or sugar-laden foods are out of your house, then you can't reach for a can of creamed corn soup mindlessly because you're feeling tired, bored, or out of sorts. You'll have to tune in to your body and consciously decide if you are physically hungry, and if so what your body actually needs.

There is a huge difference between reaching for a food once in a while and having the same food be part of your daily regime. It's the behaviors you repeat consistently over time—the ones that become habitual—that shape the quality of your life. It's the behaviors that you choose day-in and day-out that create momentum and fashion the big picture of your life.

So if you happen to be visiting your Aunt Mabel, who only offers you cream of corn soup with Italian bread—and you are hungry—then you can go ahead and eat it, knowing that this is not a habit, but a deviation from the healthful way you typically eat as a result of outer circumstances. You can feel confident and have the trust in yourself that even though the soup and bread taste good and you thoroughly enjoy them, you won't subject your body to these types of foods on a consistent basis. There comes a point when you can't go back to your old way of eating because you know too much. You become too self-aware. You see and feel beyond the "delicious" taste of highly processed foods to understand that such sweet tastes are a setup for food addiction and misery. You know that the sooner you return to eating water-rich foods, with healthy fat, protein, and complex carbohydrates in full balance, the easier it is and the better you feel on every level.

Unfortunately, when it comes to carbohydrate addiction, each time you reach for an offender (a food high in sugar, whether it be natural or refined), you are adding a building block to an inner state of compulsively craving carbohydrates in any form. The only way to offset this and still be able to enjoy complex carbohydrates on a regular basis, without swinging the pendulum toward compulsion, is to balance your intake of the various categories of food—healthy fat, high quality protein, and complex carbohydrate—and exercise in moderation on a regular basis.

You can repeat the entire Two-Week Mega-Nutrition Cleanse as often as necessary to make permanent changes in the way you think about yourself and food. The great thing about eating in a simpler way, aside from the freedom from food cravings itself, is that it helps you to appreciate the foods that you are eating so much more. There is no more guilt associated with food. Your tastes begin to change, and you prefer the selections that nourish you, sustain you, and bring you life.

This becomes so much easier when you understand that processed foods are so "tempting" because they are very skillfully being peddled by a greedy manipulative food industry that is in bed with the diet and pharmaceutical industries. My clients ask me, "What if I can't be hypnotized?" The truth is these booming industries have already created a mass hypnosis on this planet. They have taken harmful foods and substances and linked them to the very emotions we all want to feel—love, acceptance, camaraderie and happiness—thus creating desire. Once we act on that desire by consuming the food or drink, we are even more in their net because now we get hooked on the "delicious" chemical tastes they have masterfully put together, in an effort to keep us coming back, begging for more. The great news is that as individuals we can choose to not get caught in the false pleasure they are promising, by choosing what we focus on, and reminding ourselves of what's true and our own inner power.

· ·

EXERCISE: PUTTING YOUR FOOD URGES ON PAPER

To increase your ability to observe yourself, begin to carry a small notebook around with you. Every time you have the urge to binge or eat foods that you know are harmful to you, write it down, whether you act on your urge or not. First write down the outer situation that is occurring. Then jot down your thoughts about this trigger—what it means to you. Now look inside to see what your true need is. Take time to give yourself what you need. Change your self-talk from being punishing or judging to being loving and supportive. Imagine yourself giving to yourself in a deep, nurturing way.

Using the Tools

Aside from eating in a balanced way, remember to keep yourself centered through regular practice of the Break-Your-Craving-State Technique and the deep breathing and movement that are part of it. By getting into the habit of changing your physiology, including posture and breathing—while remaining conscious of your emotional and mental state—you can begin to make new, healthier choices about how you respond to your internal and external cues.

The breathing exercises in Chapter 5 can help you to achieve a much more resourceful state of consciousness than you may typically be accustomed to. In fact, one of the most common methods of achieving a hypnotic state or entering into deep meditation is through the breath. The breath is the bridge between the outer, physical world, maintaining our life, and the inner realms where our greatest strengths lie.

Regular power breathing will not only fill you up with oxygen and help to eliminate any toxic buildup in your system, but it will also help you to discover the greater power that resides within. Be aware of your tendency to revert back to shallow breathing. The more you incorporate the deep breathing—coupled with physical movement that you enjoy—the more you will naturally charge up your energy level and boost your mental clarity and vitality.

By practicing the deep breathing and by centering yourself with positive, nurturing imagery you can eliminate the negative effects of stress. There is a big difference between passively relaxing, as when you watch TV, and actively relaxing, where you actually turn on and engage the deep relaxation system in the body. This relaxation response, awakened through breathing meditation, visualization, and self-hypnosis, deeply rejuvenates you, soothes your nervous system, and feeds your being, even more than sleep.

It activates your parasympathetic nervous system and subdues the sympathetic fight or flight response. When the parasympathetic nervous system is engaged, all systems of your body normalize and optimize. Your blood vessels dilate, sending more blood and oxygen to your periphery. Your heart rate slows down and your muscles relax. Your brain waves slow from the chattering beta level to the alpha level, activating tranquility and serenity within. With regular practice, you can learn to truly feel the calm in the midst of the storm and live in that place.

Remember that up until now your addiction has been filling needs for you. Now that you have new options for filling those needs—both your physical need for nutrients and your psychological and spiritual need for love, inner peace, safety, and connection—you can look forward to shedding your old, unproductive eating habits of the past.

What a thrill it is to find your taste for food changing so that you automatically begin to prefer and select delicious, whole foods that nourish your body and sustain your life. At the same time, you'll continue to feel the relief of being turned off to those processed, empty-calorie items that are harmful to you. You can truly begin to look forward to your new sugar-free, addiction-free, life and the greater future that you are creating for yourself. Say yes to this new destiny! Welcome the true longing of your spirit to feel healthy, whole, and vital!

INDEX

Made in the USA
Columbia, SC
24 August 2019